THE COMPLETE 2021 OPTAVIA DIET COOKBOOK

THE EASIEST GUIDE TO LOSE WEIGHT PERMANENTLY. BASES, BENEFITS, PRIMARY STAGES OF THIS DIET, AND MORE. INCLUDING HEALTHY AND DELICIOUS RECIPES FOR BUSY PEOPLE

TABLE OF CONTENTS

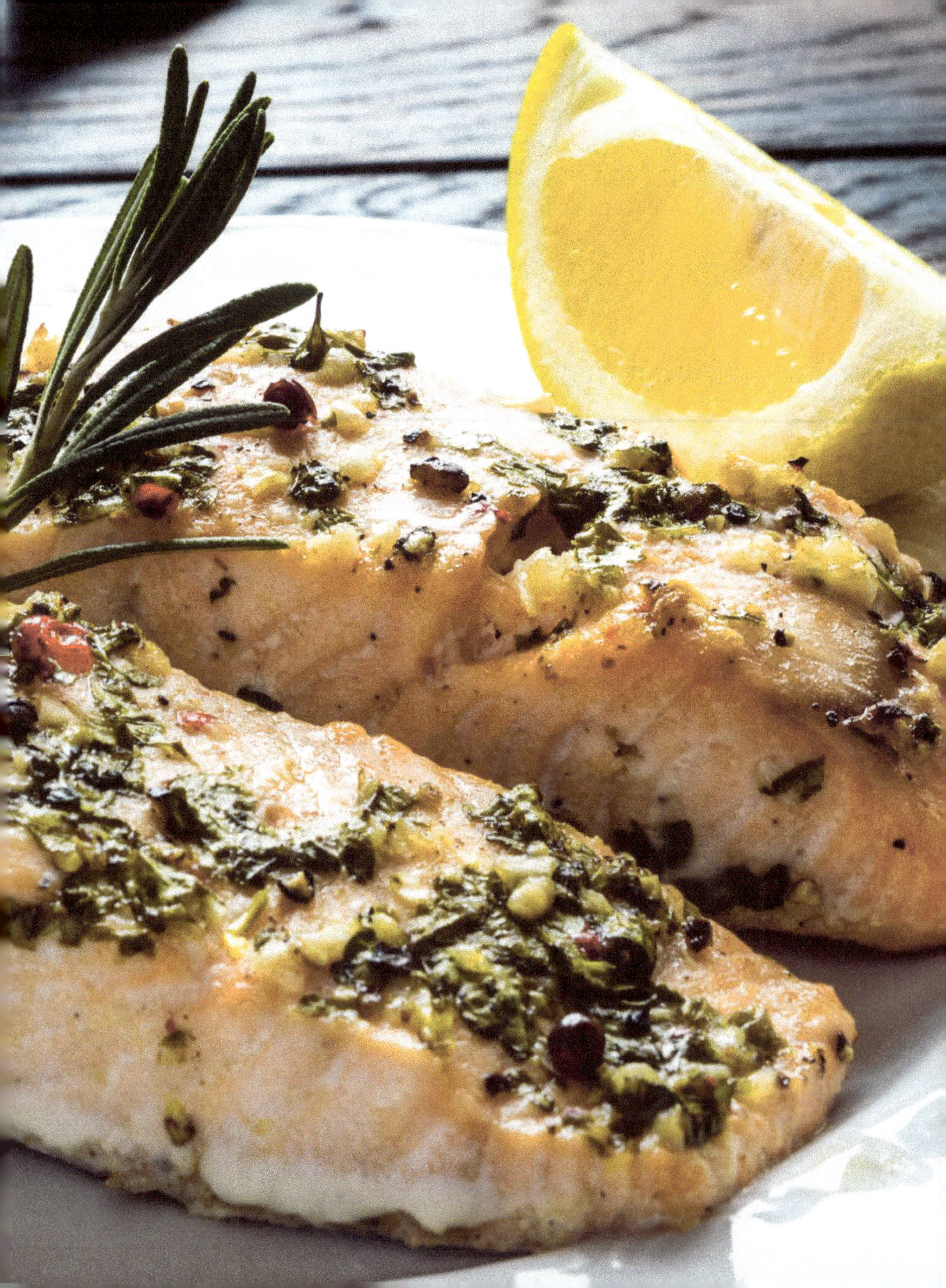

INTRODUCTION

Optavia diet was developed to help people lose weight and fat by cutting their carbs and calories through portion-controlled snacks and meals.

The 5&1 plan is not going beyond 800–1,000 calories per day for a maximum number of 6 portioned-controlled meals.

Studies of people that have taken this diet plan show that it can be beneficial in achieving weight loss than traditional calorie-restricted diets. A 16-week study conducted on 198 people who are obese or overweight shows that those who took Optavia's 5&1 plan were able to lower their weight significantly as well as their waist circumference and their fat levels. However, those in the control group were not able to achieve such a level of success.

Specifically, the result shows that those that engage in the 5&1 plan were able to shed over 5.7% of their weight. Moreover, 28.1% of these people were able to lose 10% of this. Hence, this diet plan can guarantee a 5–10% weight loss with a lower risk of type 2 diabetes and heart disease.

The record has it that those on the 5&1 diet plan and took part in up to 75% of their coaching sessions can shed twice as much weight than those that participate in fewer coaching sessions. Hence, this shows that if you take the diet plan, the coaching session is crucial as it is one of the determinants for your successful goals.

In essence, the Optavia diet is a useful tool in losing weight on a short-term basis, which is evident since you will be consuming just about half of the recommended calories for adults. However, there is research made on the long-term effectiveness of this diet plan, although there is not yet, an effective and sustainable one at the time of writing this book.

CHAPTER 1. BENEFITS OF THE OPTAVIA DIET

The Optavia diet has many benefits that can be achieved by an individual when practiced according to its "stern" guidelines. Some of the services are:

Optavia Diet Is Easy to Follow

- **Taking the diet is very easy as it relies mainly on prepackaged fuelling, and out of all of the six meals, you will need to take per day while on the 5&1 plan, you will only need to cook only 1 of the meals.**
- **An example of meals and records to help you maintain the diet.**
- **You can only cook a maximum of 1–3 lean and green meals daily based on the type of plan you are taking, and these meals are straightforward to make. They will give you a list of food options and specific recipes where you can choose.**
- **Those that are engaged and too busy to cook but wish to take on the Optavia diet plan can still practice it with ease as there is an option of buying packaged meals, these are referred to as Flavors of Home; this can replace the lean and green meals.**

Ability to Improve Blood Pressure

- **The Optavia diet program can improve participants' blood pressure since low sodium consumption and weight loss.**
- **Most Optavia meals will not give you more than 2,300mg of sodium daily.**
- **Several health organizations such as the American Heart Association, Institute of Medicine, and the United States Department of Agriculture (USDA) have already given recommendations. They advised on consuming less than 2,300mg of sodium daily since higher sodium consumption can increase the probability of growing heart disease and high blood pressure in salt-sensitive people.**

Ongoing Support

- **Once you subscribe to the Optavia program, you will have access to the coach assigned to you throughout the cause. It is valid for whichever plan you put up for, either for weight maintenance or loss.**

- **The numerous coaching sessions associated with the program have shown to enhance weight loss among the participants significantly.**

Another lifestyle coach support that has been effective in achieving significant weight loss and maintenance, the flexibility of the meal plans, which makes it easy to follow, the ability to lose excess weight and fats in few, and much more. When you subscribe to the Optavia diet program, there are a lot of benefits you will gain.

CHAPTER 2.
BASICS OF OPTAVIA DIET

Why Is This Diet Easy to Follow?

When embarking on any new diet regimen, you may experience some difficulties along the way. Below are the reasons why this diet regimen is considered as the easiest to follow among all commercial diet regimens:

- Eating out can be challenging but still possible: If you love eating out, you can download Optavia's dining out guide. It comes with tips on how to navigate buffets, order beverages, and choose condiments. Aside from following the manual, you can also ask the chef to make substitutions for the ingredients used in cooking your food. For instance, you can ask the chef to serve no more than 7 ounces of steak and serve it with steamed broccoli instead of baked potatoes.
- Pick or opt for lean and green foods that have high fullness index: Eat foods that contain high protein and fiber content as they can keep you full for more extended periods. Many nutrition experts highlight the importance of satiety when it comes to weight loss.

Do I Need Advice from Doctors or Nutritionist?

You should have access to a knowledgeable coach. If you follow the Optavia Diet plan, you should have access to knowledgeable coaches and become a member of an organization that will give you access to support calls and events. You also have a standby nutrition support team that can answer your questions.

Optavia Diet Plans FAQs

You may have some questions about the Optavia Diet Plan. Below are some of the common FAQs that people ask about this diet regimen:

1. Which program is right for me?

Optavia offers a wide variety of programs that are designed to improve health and well-being. Choosing the right one is easy as these diet plans are developed for different individuals and their needs. But, if you are still not convinced which diet plan to follow, you can always get in touch with an Optavia coach to learn about the many options that you have.

2. Is it okay for me to skip fuelling?

Fuelings is very important as it is specifically formulated with the right balance of macronutrients (carbohydrates, fats, and protein). Proper fueling can help promote an efficient fat-burning state so that people lose fat without losing their energy. If you skip it, you might miss out on these crucial nutrients, including your daily dose of vitamins and minerals. Now, if you accidentally forget it within 24 hours, it is vital to double up so that you don't miss the nutrition provided by your fuelling.

3. Which plan is best for my level of fitness?

Exercise can lead to lifelong transformation. It is the reason why the specific Optavia Diet plan is designed for people who have different activity levels. Active adults who engage in 45 minutes of light to moderate exercise can benefit from the 5&1. Always talk with your coach on which plan is great for your age and activity level.

4. Can I rearrange my fuelling, primarily if I work on long days or night duty?

Yes. You can change the schedule of your fuelling, depending on your agenda. What is important is that you consume your fuelling and lean and green meals within 24 hours. So, whether you work at night or on regular hours, make sure that you finish it every two, or if you want 3 hours throughout the time, you are awake.

5. How often should I eat my meals?

The Optavia Diet plan teaches you the habit of eating healthy. You are encouraged to eat six small meals daily. As mentioned earlier, you are encouraged to eat every two to three hours from your waking time. Thus, start your day with fuelling and eat your lean and green meals during the day. It is recommended that you eat your first meal within an hour of waking to ensure optimal blood sugar. It is also a good strategy for hunger control.

CHAPTER 3. PRIMARY STAGES OF THE DIET AND MORE INFO ABOUT OPTAVIA DIET

Notwithstanding the arrangement you pick, you start by having a telephone discussion with a mentor to help figure out which Optavia plan to follow, set weight reduction objectives, and acclimate yourself with the program.

Beginning Stages

For weight reduction, the vast majority start with the Optimal Weight 5&1 Plan. An 800–1,000 calorie routine said to assist you with dropping 12 pounds (5.4 kg) for more than 12 weeks.

On this arrangement, you eat 5 Optavia Fuelings and 1 Lean and Green supper every day. You're intended to eat one supper each 2–3 hours and fuse 30 minutes of moderate exercise most days of the week.

Altogether, the fuelings and feast give close to 100 grams of carbs every day.

You request these suppers from your mentor's site, as Optavia mentors get paid on commission.

Lean and Green suppers are intended to be high in protein and low in carbs. One dinner offers 5–7 ounces (145–200 grams) of cooked lean protein, three servings of non-dull vegetables, and up to 2 servings of solid fats.

This arrangement additionally incorporates one discretionary nibble for each day, which must be endorsed by your mentor. Plan-endorsed snacks include three celery sticks, 1/2 cup (60 grams) of without sugar gelatin, or 1/2 ounce (14 grams) of nuts.

The program likewise incorporates a feasting out guide that discloses how to arrange a Lean and Green supper with your preferred coffee. Remember that liquor is firmly disheartened on the 5&1 Plan.

Support Stage

When you arrive at your ideal weight, you enter a 6-week change stage, which includes gradually expanding calories to close to 1,550 calories for each day and mixing it up of foods, including entire grains, organic products, and low-fat dairy.

Following a month and a half, you're intended to move onto the Optimal Health 3&3 Plan, which incorporates 3 Lean and Green dinners and 3 Fuelings every day, in addition to proceeded Optavia training.

The individuals who experience supported accomplishment on the program have the choice to get prepared as an Optavia mentor.

Would Optavia Diet Help You With Shedding Pounds?

The Optavia diet is intended to assist individuals with getting thinner and fat by diminishing calories and carbs through part-controlled dinners and tidbits.

The 5&1 arrangement limits calories to 800–1,000 calories each day partitioned between 6 divided controlled meals.

While the examination is blended, a few investigations have indicated more prominent weight reduction with full or halfway meal supplanting plans contrasted and customary calorie-confined eating regimens.

Studies likewise uncover that lessening by and massive calorie admission is viable for weight and fat misfortune—as are low carb, at any rate, temporarily.

A 16-week concentrate in 198 individuals with abundance weight or stoutness found that those on Optavia's 5&1 Plan had fundamentally lower weight, fat levels, and abdomen periphery, contrasted, and the benchmark group.

With 28.1% of members losing over 10%. It may recommend extra advantages, as research partners reduce weight by 5–10% with a diminished danger of coronary illness and type 2 diabetes.

The one-on-one instructing might be useful too.

A similar report found that people on the 5&1 eating regimen who finished in any event 75% of the training meetings lost more than twice as much weight as the individuals who partook in fewer meetings.

No different, a few various examinations exhibit a massive improvement in short-and long-haul weight reduction and diet adherence in programs that incorporate progressing training.

Presently, no examinations have analyzed the drawn-out aftereffects of the Optavia diet. An analysis of a comparative Medifast plan noticed that solitary 25% of members kept up the eating routine for as long as one year.

Another test gave some weight to recover during the weight support stage following the 5&1 Medifast diet.

The main contrast between the 5&1 Medifast diet and the 5&1 Optavia Plan is that Optavia incorporates instructing.

In general, more research is expected to survey the Optavia diet's drawn-out viability.

Other Potential Advantages

The Optavia diet has extra advantages that may support weight reduction and by and large health.

- **Simple to follow**

As the eating routine generally depends on prepackaged Fuelings, you're just answerable for preparing one feast every day on the 5&1 Plan.

Besides, each arrangement accompanies supper logs, and test dinner intends to make it simpler to follow.

While you're urged to cook 1–3 Lean and Green dinners every day, contingent upon the arrangement, they're easy to make—as the program incorporates detailed plans and a rundown of food choices.

Besides, the individuals who aren't interested in preparing meals can purchase dinner packages called Flavors of Homes.

- **May improve circulatory strain**

Optavia projects may help improve circulatory strain through weight reduction and restricted sodium admission.

While the Optavia diet has not been explicitly investigated, a 40-week study of 90 overweight people in a comparable Medifast program revealed a decrease in blood pressure.

Also, all Optavia dinner plans are intended to give under 2,300 mg of sodium for each day—even though it's dependent upon you to pick low sodium choices for Lean and Green suppers.

That is because higher sodium admission is connected to an expanded danger of hypertension and coronary illness in salt-touchy people.

- **Offers progressing support**

Optavia's health mentors are accessible all through weight reduction and upkeep programs.

As noted above, one examination found a massive connection between the number of training meetings on the Optavia 5&1 Plan and improved weight reduction.

Moreover, this plan suggests that having a mentor or advisor may help in the long-run.

CHAPTER 4.
A DEEPER LOOK INTO THE OPTAVIA DIET

The Optavia Diet encourages people to limit the number of calories that they should take daily. To make this possible, dieters are motivated to choose healthier food items and meal replacements. But unlike other types of commercial diet regimens, the Optavia Diet comes in three different variations that one can choose according to their needs.

Various Optavia Diet Plans

- **5&1 Optavia diet plan: This is the most common version of the Optavia Diet. This one includes consuming five pre packed meals from them and one home-made balanced dinner.**
- **4&2&1 Optavia diet plan: This diet plan is designed for people who want to have flexibility while following this regimen. Under this program, dieters are encouraged to eat more calories and have more flexible food choices. It means that they can finish four pre packed Optimal Health Fuelings food, three home-cooked meals from the Lean and Green, and one snack daily.**
- **5&2&2 Optavia diet plan: This diet plan is perfect for individuals who prefer to have a flexible one to achieve a healthy weight. It is recommended for a wide variety of people. Under this diet regimen, dieters must eat five fuelling, two lean and green meals, and two healthy snacks.**
- **3&3 Optavia diet plan: This diet plan is created for people who have moderate weight problems and merely want to maintain a healthy body. Under this diet plan, dieters are encouraged to consume three prepackaged Optimal Health Fuelings and three home-cooked meals.**
- **Optavia for nursing mothers: This diet regimen is designed for nursing mothers with babies of at least two months old. Aside from supporting breastfeeding mothers, it also encourages gradual weight loss.**
- **Optavia for diabetes: This Optavia Diet plan is designed for people who have type 1 and type 2 diabetes. The meal plans are developed so that dieters consume more green and lean meals, depending on their needs and condition.**

- **Optavia for gout: This diet regimen incorporates a balance of low in purines and moderate in protein.**
- **Optavia for seniors (65 years and older): this is designed for seniors. The Optavia Diet plan has some variations following the components of fuelings, depending on the needs and activities of the senior dieters.**
- **Optavia for teen boys and for teen girls (13–18 years old): Designed for active teens, the Optavia for Teens Boys and Optavia for Teens Girls provide the right nutrition to growing teens.**

Regardless of which type of Optavia Diet plan you choose, you must talk with someone to coach you. He will assist you in determining which method is right for you based on your individual goals. It is to ensure that you get the most out of the program you have chosen.

How to Start This Diet

The Optavia Diet is comprised of different phases. A certified coach will educate you on the steps that you need to undertake if you want to follow this regimen. Considering those people who are new to this diet, below are some of the matters that you need to know when starting with this diet regimen.

How to Manage This Diet

During this phase, people are encouraged to consume 800 to 1,000 calories to help you shed off at least 12 pounds within the next 12 weeks. For instance, if you are following the 5&1 Optavia Diet Plan, then you need to eat one meal every 2 or 3 hours and include a 30-minute moderate workout most days of your week. You need to consume not more than 100 grams of carbs daily during this phase.

Further, consuming the Lean and Green meals are highly encouraged. It involves eating 5 to 7 ounces of cooked lean proteins and three servings of non-starchy vegetables, and two servings of healthy fats. This phase also encourages the dieter to include one optional snack per day, such as ½-cup sugar-free gelatin, three celery sticks, and 12 ounces nuts. Aside from these things, below are other things that you need to remember when following this phase:

Make sure that the portion size recommendations are for cooked weight and not the raw one of your ingredients.

Opt for meals that are baked, grilled, broiled, or poached. Avoid frying foods, as this will increase your calorie intake.

You need to consume fish that are rich in Omega-3 fatty acids, at least two servings. These include fishes like tuna, salmon, trout, mackerel, herring, and other cold-water fishes.

Choose meatless alternatives like tofu and tempeh.

Follow the program even when you are dining out. Keep in mind that drinking alcohol is discouraged when following this plan.

How to Maintain the Desired Results

When you reach your weight goals, the next phase is the transition stage. It is a 6-week stage that involves increasing your calorie intake to 1,550 per day. It is also when you can add more varieties into your meal, such as whole grains, low-fat dairy, and fruits.

After six weeks, you can now move into the 3&3 Optavia Diet plan, so you must eat three Lean and Green meals and 3 Fueling foods.

CHAPTER 5. ADAPTATION OF THE OPTAVIA DIET: PROS AND CONS

Adaptation

The Optavia diet depends on restrictive meals substitution items and carefully calorie-controlled arranged suppers, so there's very little space for change.

The 5 and 1 plan limits calories to as low as 800–1000 every day, so it's not recommended to pregnant women or people who do a lot of exercises.

Extraordinary calorie limitation can cause exhaustion, mind haze, cerebral pains, or menstrual changes. Al things considered, the 5 and 1 alternative ought to be not utilized long haul.

Be that as it may, the 3, 2, or 1 elegant family plan between 1100 and 2500 calories each day and may be suitable for a more extended period.

Pros

The Optavia Diet may be a solid match for you on the off chance that you need a diet plan that is clear and simple to follow, which will assist you with getting in shape rapidly and offers worked in social help.

- *Bundled items offer comfort*

Optavia's shakes, soups, and other diet substitutes for Optavia are legitimately important—a degree of comfort that numerous diets don't offer.

Though you need to search for your elements for "lean and green" meals, the home conveyance choice for Optavia's "fuelling" spares time and vitality.

The moment the items reached you, they are phenomenal snatch and-go suppers.

- *Accomplishes rapid weight loss*

Most individuals require around 1600 to 3000 calories each day to keep up their weight. They were limiting that number to as low as 800 ensure weight loss for a large number of people.

Optavia's 5 and 1 plan is designed for rapid weight loss, making it a healthy choice for somebody with a clinical motivation to shed pounds quickly.

- ***Wipes out the burden of guessing***

We find that the most challenging piece of dieting is the psychological effort needed to think, plan, and cook.

Optavia reduces the pressure of feast planning and "choice exhaustion" by giving the clients the needed nourishment with "fuelling" and rules for "lean and green" suppers.

- ***Offers social help***

Social help is a crucial part of achievement with any weight loss plan. Optavia's training project and gathering calls give worked in consolation and backing for clients.

Cons

There is other some potential drawbacks to Optavia's plan, which are as follows:

- ***High monthly cost***

Optavia's expense can be an obstacle for imminent clients.

The 5 and 1 plan costs from $350 to $425 for 119 servings. (Around three weeks of meal substitutions).

While you are considering the monthly cost of this diet, remember to keep in mind that you need money for your "lean and green" meals.

- ***Incorporates a large number of foods that Undergoes a process***

Though Optavia's "fuelling" is designed with compatible supplements, they're still irrefutably prepared nourishments, which might be a mood killer for specific clients.

Research has shown that consuming a large amount of manipulated food can effectively affect one's well-being, so this part of the diet plan can be burdensome.

- ***Weight loss might be impractical***

One test recognizable to anybody on a careful nutritional plan is deciding how to keep weight loss once they've finished the program.

The equivalent goes for Optavia's program. At the point when clients return to eating ordinary suppers rather than the plan's meal substitutions, they may find that the weight they lost is immediately recovered.

CHAPTER 6. CALORIE RESTRICTION IMPACT

Even though Optavia's eating routine emphasizes eating during the day, every one of its "fuelling" just gives 110 calories. "Lean and green" foods are additionally low in calories.

At the point when you're eating fewer calories, all in all, you may discover the arrangement leaves you ravenous and unsatisfied. You may likewise feel even more effectively exhausted and even crabby.

Weariness and Isolation at Mealtimes

Optavia's dependence on meal substitutions can meddle with the social parts of getting ready and eating food.

Clients may think that it's clumsy or baffling to have a shake or bar at family supper time or when feasting out with companions.

How It Compares With Others

The Optavia Diet can be more viable for fast weight reduction than different plans, basically because of the limited number of calories its fuelling and "lean and green" meals give.

U.S. News and World Report positioned Optavia as the number two best eating routine for quick weight reduction (along with Atkins, Keto, and Weight Watchers). In 2019, it ranked this diet 31st among the best diets overall and gave it a score of 2.7/5.

Optavia requires less "mental acrobatic" than contenders like Weight Watchers (for which you need to gain proficiency with an arrangement of focuses) or Keto (for which you should intently follow and evaluate macronutrients).

Optavia's instructing segment is like Weight Watchers and Jenny Craig, the two of which urge members to select in for meetups to get social help.

The exceptionally handled nature of most nourishments you'll eat on the Optavia diet can be a drawback contrasted with the variety of new entire nourishments you can eat on increasingly independently directed plans, for example, Atkins.

Medifast additionally says its dinners have a high "completion file," which means the high protein and fiber substance should keep you feeling more. In the 2010 Nutrition Journal study, analysts revealed no striking contrasts in satiety between Medifast and different healthy foods, either in the post-meal period or in the overall totality. The Diabetes Educator, moreover, found no critical differences in dietary cravings. Livelihood specialists emphasize the meaning of satiety.

Medifast items probably won't win food rivalries. Be that as it may, a Medifast agent says the organization gets its things through a tasting board before making them accessible and continually screens client criticism, growing more top choices and ending the duds. Optavia fuelings don't contain artificial colors, flavors, or sugars.

CHAPTER 7: SMOOTHIES AND BREAKFASTS

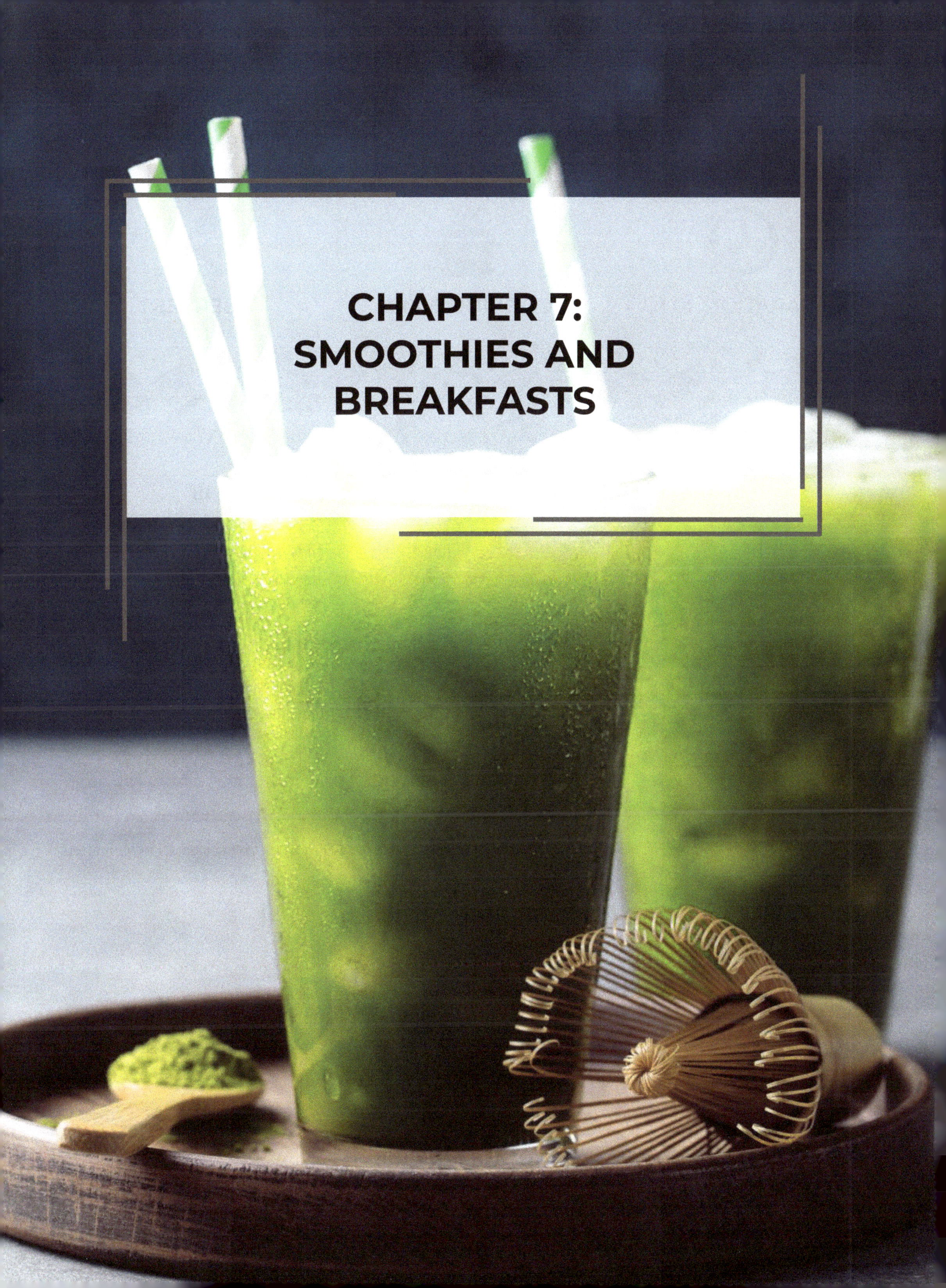

1. PROTEIN OATCAKES

PREPARATION: 10 MIN

COOKING: 5 MIN

SERVES:1

INGREDIENTS

- 70g oatmeal
- 15g protein
- 1 egg white
- ½ cup water
- ½ teaspoon cinnamon
- 60g curd
- 1 teaspoon cacao powder
- 15g sugar

DIRECTIONS

1. Mix the oatmeal, protein, egg white, and water in a bowl.
2. Preheat a saucepan to medium heat.
3. Place the mixture into the saucepan.
4. While waiting, prepare the topping by mixing the curd, cinnamon, and sugar in a second bowl.
5. Remove the oatcake from the saucepan when it becomes golden-brown.
6. Serve on a plate.
7. Add the topping and cocoa powder.

Nutritions: *Calories: 440, Protein: 1.1g, Fiber: 0.8g, Carbohydrates: 6.1g*

2. ORANGE RICOTTA PANCAKES

PREPARATION: 10 MIN

COOKING: 5 MIN

SERVES: 1

INGREDIENTS

- ¾ cup all-purpose flour
- ½ tablespoon baking powder
- 2 teaspoons sugar
- ½ teaspoon salt
- 3 separated eggs
- 1 cup fresh ricotta
- ¾ cup whole milk
- ½ teaspoon pure vanilla extract
- 1 large ripe orange

DIRECTIONS

1. Mix the flour, baking powder, sugar in a large bowl.
2. Add a pinch of salt.
3. In a separate bowl, whisk egg yolk, ricotta, milk, orange zest, and orange juice.
4. Add some vanilla extract for additional flavor.
5. Followed by the dry ingredients to the ricotta mixture and mix adequately.
6. Stir the egg white in a different bowl, and then gently fold it in the ricotta mixture.
7. Preheat saucepan to medium heat and brush with some butter until evenly spread.
8. Use a measuring cup to drop the batter onto the saucepan, ensure the pan is not crowded.
9. Allow cooking for 2 minutes.
10. Flip the food when you notice the edges begin to set, and bubbles form in the center.
11. Cook the meat for another 1 to 2 minutes.
12. Serve with any toppings of your choice.

Nutritions: *Calories: 160, Fat: 10g, Carbohydrate: 28g, Protein: 6g*

3. ASIAN SCRAMBLED EGG

PREPARATION: 10 MIN

COOKING: 10 MIN

SERVES: 1

INGREDIENTS

- 1 large egg
- 1/2 teaspoons light soy sauce
- 1/8 teaspoon white pepper
- 1 tablespoon vegetable oil

DIRECTIONS

1. Beat the eggs in a bowl.
2. To the beaten egg, add soy sauce, one-teaspoon vegetable oil, and pepper.
3. Preheat a saucepan on high heat.
4. Add the two tablespoons oil to the saucepan.
5. Then add the mixture of the beaten egg.
6. The edges will begin to cook.
7. Lessen the heat to medium and carefully scramble the eggs.
8. Turn off heat and transfer into a bowl.
9. Serve hot and enjoy

Nutritions: *Calories: 200, Fat: 6.7g, Protein: 6.1g, Carbohydrates: 1g*

4. ARTICHOKE FRITTATAS

PREPARATION: 10 MIN

COOKING: 20 MIN

SERVES: 1

INGREDIENTS

- 2.5 oz. dry spinach
- 1/4 red bell pepper
- Artichoke (drain the liquid)
- Green onions
- Dried tomatoes
- Two eggs
- Italian seasoning
- Salt
- Pepper

DIRECTIONS

1. Preheat oven to medium heat.
2. Brush a bit of oil on the cast-iron skillet.
3. Mix all the vegetables.
4. Add some seasoning.
5. Spread the vegetables evenly in the pan.
6. Whisk the eggs and add some milk.
7. Add some salt and pepper.
8. Mix in some cheese (helps to make it fluffier).
9. Pour the egg mixture in the saucepan.
10. Place the pan inside the oven for about 30 minutes.
11. Enjoy!

Nutritions: *Calories: 160, Protein: 7g, Carbohydrates: 4g, Fat: 3.5g*

5. CHOCOLATE SWEET POTATO PUDDING

PREPARATION: 5 MIN

COOKING: 2 MIN

SERVES: 1

INGREDIENTS

- 2 well-cooked sweet potatoes
- 2 tablespoons cocoa powder
- 2 tablespoons maple syrup
- ¼ cups plant-based milk (for example, almond milk)
- ¼ tablespoons salt
- ¼ tablespoons vanilla extract

DIRECTIONS

1. Inside the food processor, put all the ingredients.
2. Blend thoroughly for about 30 seconds to 1 minute.
3. Voilà!

Nutritions: *Calories: 200, Fat: 1.5g, Carbohydrates: 23.4g, Fiber: 1.3g*

6. PEANUT BUTTER AND PROTEIN PANCAKE

PREPARATION: 10 MIN

COOKING: 15 MIN

SERVES: 1

INGREDIENTS

- ½ cup oat flour
- ½ cup gluten-free chocolate pancake mix
- ½ cup almond milk
- 1 egg
- 1 tablespoon coconut water
- 1 tablespoon peanut butter
- Fresh fruits slices

DIRECTIONS

1. Preheat a saucepan to medium heat.
2. Mix the flour and the pancake mix in a mixing bowl.
3. Mix the almond milk and eggs with coconut water in another bowl.
4. Mix the dry and wet ingredients thoroughly to form a delicate batter.
5. Spray the preheated saucepan with some coconut oil.
6. Put the batter into the saucepan with a measuring cup and allow it to cook for a few minutes.
7. Allow to cool and top with peanut butter and fresh fruit slices.

Nutritions: *Calories: 380, Protein: 22g, Carbohydrates: 16g*

7. ZUCCHINI FRITTATA

PREPARATION: 20 MIN

COOKING: 20 MIN

SERVES: 1

INGREDIENTS

- 2 large zucchinis
- 1½ teaspoon of salt
- 2 eggs
- ½ cup chopped green onions
- 1 cup flour
- ½ teaspoon of black pepper
- 1 teaspoon of baking powder
- 2 tablespoons of oil

DIRECTIONS

1. Wash the two zucchinis.
2. Cut off the zucchinis on its ends and grate them in a large mixing bowl.
3. Stir in 1 teaspoon of salt and set aside for about 10 minutes (The salt helps to draw out the water from the zucchinis).
4. Squeeze dry the grated zucchinis to remove as much water as possible.
5. Then followed by the two whole eggs and the chopped green onions.
6. In a bowl, mix a cup flour, ½ teaspoon of salt, ½ teaspoon of black pepper, and one teaspoon of baking powder.
7. Next, pour the contents of the smaller bowl to those of the larger bowl containing the grated zucchinis.
8. Stir them all together and make sure they are well mixed.
9. Preheat a saucepan to medium temperature and add two tablespoons of oil.
10. Add the zucchini mixture a heaping tablespoonful at a time.
11. Sauté the mixture for about 4 minutes on each side, to achieve a golden-brown color.
12. Add more oil to the pan if needed.
13. Serve and enjoy!

Nutritions: *Calories: 200, Protein: 7g, Carbohydrates: 4g, Fat: 3.5g*

8. TEX-MEX TOFU BREAKFAST TACOS

PREPARATION: 10 MIN

COOKING: 15 MIN

SERVES: 1

INGREDIENTS

- 8 oz. firm tofu
- 1 cup well-cooked black bean
- 1/4 red onion
- 1 cup fresh coriander
- 1 ripe avocado
- 1/2 cup salsa
- 1 medium-sized lime
- 5 whole corn tortillas
- 1/2 teaspoon garlic powder
- 1/2 teaspoon chili powder
- 1/8 teaspoon of sea salt
- 1 tablespoon salsa
- 1 tablespoon water

DIRECTIONS

1. Dice the red onions, avocados, coriander, and keep in separate bowls.
2. Also, slice the limes and keep in individual bowls.
3. In a clean towel. Wrap the tofu and place under a cast-iron skillet.
4. In the meantime, heat a saucepan to medium heat.
5. Cook the black beans in the saucepan, add a little amount of salt, cumin, and chili powder.
6. Then decrease the heat to a low simmer and set aside.
7. Add the tofu spices and salsa into a bowl, then add some water and set aside.
8. Heat another skillet to medium heat.
9. Pour some oil into the skillet, and then crumble the tofu into it.
10. Stir-fry for about 5 minutes until the tofu begins to brown.
11. Add some seasoning and continue to cook for about 5 to 10 minutes, and then set aside.
12. Heat the tortillas in oven to 250°F.
13. Top the tortillas with tofu scramble, avocado, salsa, coriander, black beans, and lime juice.
14. Serve immediately.

Nutritions: *Calories: 350, Fat: 6.5g, Carbohydrates: 23.6g, Protein: 21.5g*

9. MOCHA OATMEAL

PREPARATION: 5 MIN

COOKING: 10 MIN

SERVES: 1

INGREDIENTS

- 1 banana
- ½ cup oats
- 1 cup coffee
- ¼ teaspoon salt
- 1 teaspoon walnut
- ½ teaspoon cacao powder
- 1 cup milk
- Honey

DIRECTIONS

1. Preheat a saucepan to medium heat.
2. Put the oats in a saucepan.
3. Slice the banana, mash them, and add them to the oats.
4. Add coffee, walnuts, cacao powder, and salt.
5. Stir and you may want to wait for it to simmer, practically until the mixture becomes sticky inconsistency.
6. Serve in a bowl and add milk and honey as desired.
7. Enjoy!

Nutritions: *Calories: 400, Carbohydrates: 51g, Fats: 5g, Fiber: 8g*

10. BLACK AND BLUEBERRY PROTEIN SMOOTHIE

PREPARATION: 5 MIN

COOKING: 0 MIN

SERVES: 1

INGREDIENTS

- 1 cup sugar-free coconut milk (or any other plant-based milk of your choice)
- 1 scoop vanilla or natural protein powder
- 6 oz. fat-free vanilla Greek yogurt
- 2 tablespoons of milled flaxseed
- 1 cup berries (black or blue)
- 1 cup ice

DIRECTIONS

1. In the food processor, place all the ingredients.
2. Blend until smooth.
3. Pour into a cup and enjoy.

Nutritions: *Calories: 360, Fats: 1.5g, Protein: 49g, Carbohydrates: 40g*

11. SHAKE CAKE FUELING

PREPARATION: 5 MIN

COOKING: 0 MIN

SERVES: 1

INGREDIENTS

- 1 packet optavia shakes.
- ¼ teaspoon baking powder
- 2 tablespoons eggbeaters or egg whites
- 2 tablespoons water.
- Other options that are not compulsory include sweetener, reduced-fat cream cheese, ketchup

DIRECTIONS

1. Begin by preheating the oven.
2. Mix all the ingredients begin with the dry ingredients first before adding the wet ingredients.
3. After the mixture/batter is ready, pour gently into muffin cups.
4. Inside the oven, place, and bake for about 16–18minutes or until it is baked and ready. Allow it to cool completely.
5. Add additional toppings of your choice and ensure your delicious shake cake is refreshing.

Nutritions: *Calories: 896, Fat: 37g, Carbohydrate: 115g, Protein: 34g*

12. CAULIFLOWER CRUST PIZZA

PREPARATION: 15 MIN COOKING: 30-35 MIN SERVES: 1

INGREDIENTS

- 1/4 cauliflower (it should be cut into smaller portions)
- 1/16 grated parmesan cheese
- 1/2 egg
- ½ teaspoon Italian seasoning
- 1/16 teaspoon kosher salt
- 1 cups of freshly grated mozzarella
- 1/4 cup spicy pizza sauce.
- Basil leaves, for garnishing.

DIRECTIONS

1. Begin by preheating your oven while using the parchment paper to rim the baking sheet.
2. Process the cauliflower into a fine powder, and then transfer to a bowl before putting it into the microwave. Leave for about 5–6 minutes to get it soft.
3. Transfer the microwaved cauliflower to a clean and dry kitchen towel. Leave it to cool.
4. When cold, use the kitchen towel to wrap the cauliflower and then get rid of all the moisture by wringing the towel. Continue squeezing until water is gone completely.
5. Put the cauliflower, Italian seasoning, parmesan, egg, salt, and mozzarella (1 cup). Stir very well until well combined.
6. Transfer the combined mixture to the baking sheet previously prepared, pressing it into a 10-inch round shape.
7. Wait for it to bake until it becomes golden in color.
8. Take the baked crust out of the oven and use the spicy pizza sauce and mozzarella (the leftover 1 cup) to top it. Put it again inside the oven for ten more minutes until the cheese melts and looks bubbly.
9. Garnish using fresh basil leaves. You can also enjoy this with salad.

Nutritions: *Calories: 230, Fat: 8g, Carbohydrate: 28g, Protein: 6g*

13. ZUCCHINI FRITTERS

PREPARATION: 5 MIN

COOKING: 15 MIN

SERVES: 1

INGREDIENTS

- 1/4 pound grated zucchini
- 1/4 teaspoon salt
- 1/16 cup grated parmesan
- 1/16 cup flour
- 1/2 cloves minced garlic
- 1/2 tablespoon olive oil
- 1/4 large egg
- Newly ground black pepper and kosher salt to taste

DIRECTIONS

1. Put the grated zucchini into a colander over the sink.
2. Add your salt and toss it to mix properly, then leave it to settle for about 10 minutes.
3. Next, use a clean cheesecloth to drain the zucchini completely.
4. Combine drained zucchini, parmesan, garlic, flour, and the beaten egg in a large bowl, mix, and season with pepper and salt.
5. Then, pour the olive oil in a skillet applying medium-high heat.
6. Use a tablespoon to scoop batter for each fritter, put in the oil, and flatten using a spatula.
7. Allow to cook until the underside is richly golden brown, then flip over to the other side and cook.
8. Your delicious zucchini fritters are ready to be served.

Nutritions: *Calories: 105.1, Fat: 2.8g, Carbohydrate: 15.8g, Protein: 6g*

14. OPTAVIA PIZZA HACK

PREPARATION: 5-10 MIN

COOKING: 10-20 MIN

SERVES: 1

INGREDIENTS

- 1/4 fueling garlic mashed potato
- 1/2 egg whites
- 1/4 tablespoon baking powder
- 3/4 oz. reduced-fat shredded mozzarella
- 1/8 cup sliced white mushrooms
- 1/16 cup pizza sauce
- 3/4 oz. ground beef
- 1/4 sliced black olives
- You also need a sauté pan, baking sheets, and parchment paper

DIRECTIONS

1. Start by preheating the oven to 400°F.
2. Mix your baking powder and garlic potato packet.
3. Add egg whites to your mixture and stir well until it blends.
4. Line the baking sheet with parchment paper and pour the mixed batter onto it.
5. Put another parchment paper on top of the batter and spread out the batter to a 1/8-inch circle.
6. Then place another baking sheet on top; this way, the matter is between two baking sheets.
7. Place into an oven and bake for about 8 minutes until the pizza crust is golden brown.
8. For the toppings, place your ground beef in a sauté pan and fry until its brown and wash your mushrooms very well.
9. After the crust is baked, remove the top layer of parchment paper carefully to prevent the paper from sticking to the pizza crust.
10. Put your toppings on top of the crust and bake for an extra 8 minutes.
11. Once ready, slide the pizza off the parchment paper and into a plate.

Nutritions: *Calories: 478, Protein: 30g, Carbohydrates: 22g, Fats: 29g*

15. OPTAVIA BISCUIT PIZZA

PREPARATION: 5 MIN

COOKING: 15-20 MIN

SERVES: 1

INGREDIENTS

- 1/4 sachet optavia buttermilk cheddar and herb biscuit
- 1/4 tablespoon tomato sauce
- 1/4 tablespoon low-fat shredded cheese
- 1/4 table of water
- Parchment paper

DIRECTIONS

1. You may begin by preheating the oven to about 350°F.
2. Mix the biscuit and water and stir properly.
3. In the parchment paper, pour the mixture and spread it into a thin circle. Allow cooking for 10 minutes.
4. Take it out and add the tomato sauce and shredded cheese.
5. Bake it for a few more minutes.

Nutritions: *Calories: 478, Protein: 30g, Carbohydrates: 22g, Fats: 29g*

16. MINI MAC IN A BOWL

PREPARATION: 5 MIN

COOKING: 15 MIN

SERVES: 1

INGREDIENTS

- 5 oz. lean ground beef
- 2 tablespoons diced white or yellow onion.
- 1/8 teaspoon onion powder
- 1/8 teaspoon white vinegar
- 1 oz. dill pickle slices
- 1 teaspoon sesame seed
- 3 cups shredded romaine lettuce
- Cooking spray
- 2 tablespoons reduced-fat shredded cheddar cheese
- 2 tablespoons wish-bone light thousand island as dressing

DIRECTIONS

1. Place a lightly greased small skillet on fire to heat.
2. Add your onion to cook for about 2–3 minutes.
3. Next, add the beef and allow it to cook until it is brown.
4. Next, mix your vinegar and onion powder with the dressing.
5. Finally, top the lettuce with the cooked meat and sprinkle cheese on it, add your pickle slices.
6. Drizzle the mixture with the sauce and sprinkle the sesame seeds also.
7. Your mini mac in a bowl is ready for consumption.

Nutritions: *Calories: 150, Protein: 21g, Carbohydrates: 32g, Fats: 19g*

17. LEAN AND GREEN SMOOTHIE 1

PREPARATION: 5 MIN

COOKING: 0 MIN

SERVES: 1

INGREDIENTS

- 2 ½ cups of kale leaves
- ¾ cup chilled apple juice
- 1 cup cubed pineapple
- ½ cup frozen green grapes
- ½ cup chopped apple

DIRECTIONS

1. Place the pineapple, apple juice, apple, frozen seedless grapes, and kale leaves in a blender.
2. Cover and blend until it's smooth.
3. Smoothie is ready and can be garnished with halved grapes if you wish.

Nutritions: *Calories: 81, Protein: 2g, Carbohydrates: 19g, Fats: 1g*

18. LEAN AND GREEN SMOOTHIE 2

PREPARATION: 5 MIN

COOKING: 0 MIN

SERVES: 1

INGREDIENTS

- 6 kale leaves
- 2 peeled oranges
- 2 cups mango kombucha
- 2 cups chopped pineapple
- 2 cups water

DIRECTIONS

1. Break up the oranges, place in the blender.
2. Add the mango kombucha, chopped pineapple, and kale leaves into the blender.
3. Blend everything until it is smooth.
4. Smoothie is ready to be taken.

Nutritions: *Calories: 81, Protein: 2g, Carbohydrates: 19g, Fats: 1g*

19. LEAN AND GREEN CHICKEN PESTO PASTA

PREPARATION: 5 MIN   COOKING: 15 MIN   SERVES: 1

INGREDIENTS

- 3 cups raw kale leaves
- 2 tablespoon olive oil
- 2 cups fresh basil
- ¼ teaspoon salt
- 3 tablespoon lemon juice
- 3 garlic cloves
- 2 cups cooked chicken breast
- 1 cup baby spinach
- 6 oz. uncooked chicken pasta
- 3 oz. diced fresh mozzarella
- Basil leaves or red pepper flakes to garnish

DIRECTIONS

1. Start by making the pesto, add the kale, lemon juice, basil, garlic cloves, olive oil, and salt to a blender and blend until it is smooth.
2. Add pepper to taste.
3. Cook the pasta and strain off the water. Reserve ¼ cup of the liquid.
4. Get a bowl and mix everything, the cooked pasta, pesto, diced chicken, spinach, mozzarella, and the reserved pasta liquid.
5. Sprinkle the mixture with additional chopped basil or red paper flakes (optional).
6. Now your salad is ready. You may serve it warm or chilled. Also, it can be taken as a salad mix-ins or as a side dish. Leftovers should be stored in the refrigerator inside an air-tight container for 3–5 days.

Nutritions: *Calories: 244, Protein: 20.5g, Carbohydrates: 22.5g, Fats: 10g*

20. TROPICAL GREENS SMOOTHIE

PREPARATION: 5 MIN

COOKING: 0 MIN

SERVES: 1

INGREDIENTS

- 1 banana
- 1/2 large navel orange, peeled and segmented
- 1/2 cup frozen mango chunks
- 1 cup frozen spinach
- 1 celery stalk, broken into pieces
- 1 tablespoon cashew butter or almond butter
- 1/2 tablespoon spiraling
- 1/2 tablespoon ground flaxseed
- 1/2 cup unsweetened nondairy milk
- Water, for thinning (optional)

DIRECTIONS

1. In a high-speed blender or food processor, combine the bananas, orange, mango, spinach, celery, cashew butter, spiraling (if using), flaxseed, and milk.
2. Blend until creamy, adding more milk or water to thin the smoothie if too thick. Serve immediately—it is best served fresh.

Nutritions: *Calories: 391, Fat: 12g, Protein: 13g, Carbohydrates: 68g, Fiber: 13g*

21. VITAMIN C SMOOTHIE CUBES

PREPARATION: 5 MIN   COOKING: 8 HOURS TO CHILL   SERVES: 1

INGREDIENTS

- 1/8 large papaya
- 1/8 mango
- 1/4 cups chopped pineapple, fresh or frozen
- 1/8 cup raw cauliflower florets, fresh or frozen
- 1/4 large navel oranges, peeled and halved
- 1/4 large orange bell pepper stemmed, seeded, and coarsely chopped

DIRECTIONS

1. Halve the papaya and mango, remove the pits, and scoop their soft flesh into a high-speed blender.
2. Add the pineapple, cauliflower, oranges, and bell pepper. Blend until smooth.
3. Evenly divide the puree between 2 (16-compartment) ice cube trays and place them on a level surface in your freezer. Freeze for at least 8 hours.
4. The cubes can be left in the ice cube trays until use or transferred to a freezer bag. The frozen cubes are good for about three weeks in a standard freezer or up to 6 months in a chest freezer.

Nutritions: *Calories: 96, Fat: 1g, Protein: 2g, Carbohydrates: 24g, Fiber: 4g*

22. OVERNIGHT CHOCOLATE CHIA PUDDING

PREPARATION: 2 MIN COOKING: OVERNIGHT TO CHILL SERVES: 1

INGREDIENTS

- 1/8 cup chia seeds
- 1/2 cup unsweetened nondairy milk
- 1 tablespoon raw cacao powder
- 1/2 teaspoon vanilla extract
- 1/2 teaspoon pure maple syrup

DIRECTIONS

1. Stir together the chia seeds, milk, cacao powder, vanilla, and maple syrup in a large bowl. Divide between 2 (½-pint) covered glass jars or containers. Refrigerate overnight.
2. Stir before serving.

Nutritions: *Calories: 213, Fat: 10g, Protein: 9g, Carbohydrates: 20g, Fiber: 15g*

23. SLOW COOKER SAVORY BUTTERNUT SQUASH OATMEAL

PREPARATION: 15 MIN

COOKING: 6-8 H

SERVES: 1

INGREDIENTS

- 1/4 cup steel-cut oats
- 1/2 cups cubed (½-inch pieces) peeled butternut squash (freeze any leftovers after preparing a whole squash for future meals)
- 3/4 cups water
- 1/16 cup unsweetened nondairy milk
- 1/4 tablespoon chia seed
- 1/2 teaspoons yellow (mellow) miso paste
- 3/4 teaspoons ground ginger
- 1/4 tablespoon sesame seed, toasted
- 1/4 tablespoon chopped scallion, green parts only
- Shredded carrot, for serving (optional)

DIRECTIONS

1. In a slow cooker, combine the oats, butternut squash, and water.
2. Cover the slow cooker and cook on low for 6 to 8 hours, or until the squash is fork-tender. Using a potato masher or heavy spoon, roughly mash the cooked butternut squash. Stir to combine with the oats.
3. Whisk together the milk, chia seeds, miso paste, and ginger to combine in a large bowl. Stir the mixture into the oats.
4. Top your oatmeal bowl with sesame seeds and scallion for more plant-based fiber, top with shredded carrot (if using).

Nutritions: *Calories: 230, Fat: 5g, Protein: 7g, Carbohydrates: 40g, Fiber: 9g*

24. CARROT CAKE OATMEAL

PREPARATION: 10 MIN | COOKING: 15 MIN | SERVES: 1

INGREDIENTS

- 1/8 cup pecans
- 1/2 cup finely shredded carrot
- 1/4 cup old-fashioned oats
- 5/8 cups unsweetened nondairy milk
- 1/2 tablespoon pure maple syrup
- 1/2 teaspoon ground cinnamon
- 1/2 teaspoon ground ginger
- 1/8 teaspoon ground nutmeg
- 1 tablespoon chia seed

DIRECTIONS

1. Over medium-high heat in a skillet, toast the pecans for 3 to 4 minutes, often stirring, until browned and fragrant (watch closely, as they can burn quickly). Pour the pecans onto a cutting board and coarsely chop them. Set aside.
2. In an 8-quart pot over medium-high heat, combine the carrot, oats, milk, maple syrup, cinnamon, ginger, and nutmeg. When it is already boiling, reduce the heat to medium-low. Cook, uncovered, for 10 minutes, stirring occasionally.
3. Stir in the chopped pecans and chia seeds. Serve immediately.

Nutritions: *Calories: 307, Fat: 17g, Protein: 7g, Carbohydrates: 35g, Fiber: 11g*

25. SPICED SORGHUM AND BERRIES

PREPARATION: 5 MIN

COOKING: 1 H

SERVES: 1

INGREDIENTS

- 1/4 cup whole-grain sorghum
- 1/4 teaspoon ground cinnamon
- 1/4 teaspoon Chinese five-spice powder
- 3/4 cups water
- 1/4 cup unsweetened nondairy milk
- 1/4 teaspoon vanilla extract
- 1/2 tablespoons pure maple syrup
- 1/2 tablespoon chia seed
- 1/8 cup sliced almonds
- 2 cups fresh raspberries, divided

DIRECTIONS

1. Using a large pot over medium-high heat, stir together the sorghum, cinnamon, five-spice powder, and water. Wait for the water to a boil, cover the bank, and reduce the heat to medium-low. Cook for 1 hour, or until the sorghum is soft and chewy. If the sorghum grains are still hard, add another cup of water and cook for 15 minutes more.
2. Using a glass measuring cup, whisk together the milk, vanilla, and maple syrup to blend. Add the mixture to the sorghum and the chia seeds, almonds, and 1 cup of raspberries. Gently stir to combine.
3. When serving, top with the remaining 1 cup of fresh raspberries.

Cover the slow cooker and cook on low for 6 to 8 hours

Nutritions: *Calories: 289, Fat: 8g, Protein: 9g, Carbohydrates: 52g, Fiber: 10g*

26. RAW-CINNAMON-APPLE NUT BOWL

PREPARATION: 15 MIN COOKING: 1 H TO CHILL SERVES: 1

INGREDIENTS

- 1 green apple halved, seeded, and cored
- 3/4 honey crisp apples, halved, seeded, and cored
- 1/4 teaspoon freshly squeezed lemon juice
- 1 pitted medrol dates
- 1/8 teaspoon ground cinnamon
- Pinch ground nutmeg
- 1/2 tablespoons chia seeds, plus more for serving (optional)
- 1/4 tablespoon hemp seed
- 1/8 cup chopped walnuts
- Nut butter, for serving (optional)

DIRECTIONS

1. Finely dice half the green apple and honey crisp apple. With the lemon juice, store it in an airtight container while you work on the next steps.
2. Coarsely chop the remaining apples and the dates. Transfer to a food processor and add the cinnamon and nutmeg. Check it several times if it combines, then processes for 2 to 3 minutes to puree. Stir the puree into the reserved diced apples. Stir in the chia seeds (if using), hemp seeds, and walnuts. Chill for at least 1 hour. Enjoy!
3. Serve as is or top with additional chia seeds and nut butter (if using).

Nutritions: *Calories: 274, Fat: 8g, Protein: 4g, Carbohydrates: 52g, Fiber: 9g*

27. PEANUT BUTTER AND CACAO BREAKFAST QUINOA

PREPARATION: 5 MIN

COOKING: 10 MIN

SERVES: 1

INGREDIENTS

- 1/3 cup quinoa flakes
- 1/2 cup unsweetened nondairy milk
- 1/2 cup water
- 1/8 cup raw cacao powder
- 1 tablespoon natural creamy peanut butter
- 1/8 teaspoon ground cinnamon
- 1 banana, mashed
- Fresh berries of choice, for serving
- Chopped nuts of choice, for serving

DIRECTIONS

1. Using an 8-quart pot over medium-high heat, stir together the quinoa flakes, milk, water, cacao powder, peanut butter, and cinnamon. Cook and stir it until the mixture begins to simmer. Turn the heat to medium-low and cook for 3 to 5 minutes, stirring frequently.
2. Stir in the bananas and cook until hot.
3. Serve topped with fresh berries, nuts, and a splash of milk.

Nutritions: *Calories: 471, Fat: 16g, Protein: 18g, Carbohydrates: 69g, Fiber: 16g*

28. VANILLA BUCKWHEAT PORRIDGE

PREPARATION: 5 MIN

COOKING: 25 MIN

SERVES: 1

INGREDIENTS

- 1 cup water
- 1/4 cup raw buckwheat grouts
- 1/4 teaspoon ground cinnamon
- 1/4 banana, sliced
- 1/16 cup golden raisins
- 1/16 cup dried currants
- 1/16 cup sunflower seeds
- 1/2 tablespoons chia seeds
- 1/4 tablespoon hemp seed
- 1/4 tablespoon sesame seed, toasted
- 1/8 cup unsweetened nondairy milk
- 1/4 tablespoon pure maple syrup
- 1/4 teaspoon vanilla extract

DIRECTIONS

1. Boil the water in a pot. Stir in the buckwheat, cinnamon, and banana. Cook the mixture. Mixing it and wait for it to boil, then reduce the heat to medium-low. Cover the pot and cook for 15 minutes, or until the buckwheat is tender. Remove from the heat.
2. Stir in the raisins, currants, sunflower seeds, chia seeds, hemp seeds, sesame seeds, milk, maple syrup, and vanilla. Cover the pot. Wait for 10 minutes before serving.
3. Serve as is or top as desired.

Nutritions: *Calories: 353, Fat: 11g, Protein: 10g, Carbohydrates: 61g, Fiber: 10g*

29. POLENTA WITH SEARED PEARS

PREPARATION: 10 MIN

COOKING: 50 MIN

SERVES: 1

INGREDIENTS

- 1 cup water, divided, plus more as needed
- 1/2 cups coarse cornmeal
- 1 tablespoon pure maple syrup
- 1/4 tablespoon molasses
- 1/4 teaspoon ground cinnamon
- 1/2 ripe pears, cored and diced
- 1/4 cup fresh cranberries
- 1/4 teaspoon chopped fresh rosemary leaves

DIRECTIONS

1. In a pan, cook 5 cups of water to a simmer.
2. While whisking continuously to avoid clumping, slowly pour in the cornmeal. Cook, often stirring with a heavy spoon, for 30 minutes. The polenta should be thick and creamy.
3. While the polenta cooks, in a saucepan over medium heat, stir together the maple syrup, molasses, the remaining ¼-cup of water, and the cinnamon until combined. Bring it to a simmer. Add the pears and cranberries. Cook for 10 minutes, occasionally stirring, until the pears are tender and start to brown. Remove from the heat. Stir in the rosemary and let the mixture sit for 5 minutes. If it is too thick, add another ¼ cup of water and return to the heat.
4. Top with the cranberry-pear mixture.

Nutritions: *Calories: 282, Fat: 2g, Protein: 4g, Carbohydrates: 65g, Fiber: 12g*

30. BEST WHOLE WHEAT PANCAKES

PREPARATION: 10 MIN

COOKING: 20 MIN

SERVES: 1

INGREDIENTS

- 3/4 tablespoons ground flaxseed
- 2 tablespoons warm water
- 1/2 cups whole wheat pastry flour
- 1/8 cup rye flour
- 1/2 tablespoons double-acting baking powder
- 1/4 teaspoon ground cinnamon
- 1/8 teaspoon ground ginger
- 1 cup unsweetened nondairy milk
- 3/4 tablespoons pure maple syrup
- 1/4 teaspoon vanilla extract

DIRECTIONS

1. Mix the warm water and flaxseed in a large bowl. Set aside for at least 5 minutes.
2. Whisk together the pastry and rye flours, baking powder, cinnamon, and ginger to combine.
3. Whisk together the milk, maple syrup, and vanilla in a large bowl. Make use of a spatula, fold the wet ingredients into the dry ingredients. Fold in the soaked flaxseed until fully incorporated.
4. Heat a large skillet or nonstick griddle over medium-high heat. Working in batches, 3 to 4 pancakes at a time, add ¼-cup portions of batter to the hot skillet. Until golden brown, cook for 3 to 4 minutes each side or no liquid batter is visible.

Nutritions: *Calories: 301, Fat: 4g, Protein: 10g, Carbohydrates: 57g, Fiber: 10g*

31. SPICED PUMPKIN MUFFINS

PREPARATION: 15 MIN | COOKING: 20 MIN | SERVES: 1

INGREDIENTS

- 1/6 tablespoons ground flaxseed
- 1/24 cup water
- 1/8 cups whole wheat flour
- 1/6 teaspoons baking powder
- 5/6 teaspoons ground cinnamon
- 1/12 teaspoon baking soda
- 1/12 teaspoon ground ginger
- 1/16 teaspoon ground nutmeg
- 1/32 teaspoon ground cloves
- 1/6 cup pumpkin puree
- 1/12 cup pure maple syrup
- 1/24 cup unsweetened applesauce
- 1/24 cup unsweetened nondairy milk
- 1/2 teaspoons vanilla extract

DIRECTIONS

1. Preheat the oven to 350°F. Line a 12-cup metal muffin pan with parchment paper liners or use a silicone muffin pan.
2. First, mix the flaxseed and water in a large bowl then keep it aside.
3. In a medium bowl, stir together the flour, baking powder, cinnamon, baking soda, ginger, nutmeg, and cloves.
4. In a medium bowl, stir up the maple syrup, pumpkin puree, applesauce, milk, and vanilla. Crease the wet ingredients into the dry ingredients make use of a spatula.
5. Fold the soaked flaxseed into the batter until evenly combined, but do not over mix the batter, or your muffins will become dense. Spoon about ¼ cup of batter per muffin into your prepared muffin pan.
6. Bake for 18 to 20 minutes, or until a toothpick inserted into the center of a muffin comes out clean. Remove the muffins from the pan.
7. Transfer to a wire rack for cooling.
8. Store in an airtight container that is at room temperature.

Nutritions: *Calories: 115, Fat: 1g, Protein: 3g, Carbohydrates: 25g, Fiber: 3g*

32. ORANGE RESOLUTION SMOOTHIE

PREPARATION: 5 MIN

COOKING: 0 MIN

SERVES: 1

INGREDIENTS

- 1/4 cup orange juice
- 1/2 cup Greek yogurt
- 1/2 cup frozen mango chunks
- 1 banana, peeled, frozen
- 1/4 cup miniature carrots
- 1/2 cup frozen peach slices
- 1 tablespoon honey
- 1/4 cup pineapple pieces

DIRECTIONS

1. Gather all the ingredients.
2. Start a high-powered blender, and then add together every one of the ingredients into it in the order mentioned in the list.
3. Turn it on for 45 to 60 seconds or more reliant on the blender, until well blended and smooth, and then divide the smoothie between two glasses.
4. Serve straight away.

Nutritions: *Calories: 199, Total Fat: 6g, Saturated Fat: 4.5g, Carbohydrates: 34g, Fiber: 3g, Sugars: 28g, Protein: 5g*

33. SPICY CARROT, AVOCADO, AND TOMATO SMOOTHIE

PREPARATION: 5 MIN

COOKING: 0 MIN

SERVES: 1

INGREDIENTS

- 3/4 cup coconut water, unsweetened
- ½ a medium cucumber, unpeeled, chopped
- 1 medium tomato, deseeded, chopped
- 1 avocado, peeled, pitted
- 1 cup chopped romaine lettuce
- 1 medium carrot, peeled, diced
- 1 lime, peeled, halved
- 1 clove garlic, peeled
- 3/4 teaspoon sea salt
- 1/8 teaspoon cayenne pepper
- 1 tablespoon olive oil
- 1 cup ice cubes

DIRECTIONS

1. Gather all the ingredients. Add all the ingredients into it in the order cited in a blender.
2. Pulse for 45 to 60 seconds or more varying on the blender, up until well combined and smooth, and then distribute the smoothie amongst two glasses. Serve straight away.

Nutritions: *Calories: 244, Total Fat: 17g, Saturated Fat: 2.6g, Carbohydrates: 19.2g, Fiber: 9.2g, Sugars: 7.1g, Protein: 3g*

34. ZUCCHINI BREAD SMOOTHIE

PREPARATION: 5 MIN

COOKING: 0 MIN

SERVES: 1

INGREDIENTS

- 2 cups almond milk, unsweetened
- ½ cup baby spinach leaves, fresh, rinsed
- ½ cup rolled oats
- 2 cups chopped zucchini, fresh or frozen
- 1 teaspoon ground cinnamon
- 1 tablespoon maple syrup
- ¼ teaspoon ground nutmeg
- ¼ cup walnut halves
- 1 cup ice cubes

DIRECTIONS

1. Gather all the ingredients.
2. In a high-powered blender, add up all the ingredients into it in the sort cited in the list.
3. Turn it on for 45 to 60 seconds or further dependent on the blender, until well mixed and smooth, and then distribute the smoothie between two glasses.
4. Serve straight away.

Nutritions: *Calories: 317, Total Fat: 13g, Saturated Fat: 1g, Carbohydrates: 43g, Fiber: 11g, Sugars: 17g, Protein: 13g*

35. CAULIFLOWER AND BLUEBERRY SMOOTHIE

PREPARATION: 5 MIN

COOKING: 0 MIN

SERVES: 1

INGREDIENTS

- 1 cup Greek yogurt, unsweetened
- 2 tablespoons peanut butter
- 1 ¼ cup cauliflower florets, frozen
- 1 clementines, peeled
- ½ cup spinach leaves, rinsed
- 1 cup blueberries, frozen

DIRECTIONS

1. Gather all the ingredients.
2. Socket a high-powdered blender, and later combine all the components into it in the order mentioned in the ingredients list.
3. Let it blend for 45 to 60 seconds or more reliant on the blender, until properly mixed and smooth, and then divide the smoothie between two glasses.
4. Serve straight away.

Nutritions: *Calories: 323, Total Fat: 10.6g, Saturated Fat: 3.2g, Carbohydrates: 35.8g, Fiber: 9.4g, Sugars: 26.8g, Protein: 19.9g*

36. BUTTERNUT SQUASH SMOOTHIE

PREPARATION: 5 MIN

COOKING: 0 MIN

SERVES: 1

INGREDIENTS

- 2 cups almond milk, unsweetened
- ½ cup water
- 1 cup butternut squash pieces, frozen
- 2 bananas, peeled, frozen
- 1 cup raspberries, frozen
- 2 tablespoons hemp seeds
- 1 tablespoons chia seeds
- 1 teaspoon ground cinnamon
- 1/4 cup peanut butter

DIRECTIONS

1. In a high-powdered blender, add all the ingredients into it in the order in the list.
2. Turn it on for 45 to 60 seconds or further differing on the blender, until perfectly combined and smooth, and then distribute the smoothie among two glasses.
3. Serve up straight away.

Nutritions: *Calories: 520, Total Fat: 26.1g, Saturated Fat: 4.4g, Carbohydrates: 56.2g, Fiber: 15.8g, Sugars: 22.8g, Protein: 14.1g*

37. AVOCADO AND KALE SUPER FOOD SMOOTHIE

PREPARATION: 5 MIN

COOKING: 0 MIN

SERVES: 1

INGREDIENTS

- 1/2 cup almond milk, unsweetened
- 1/2 cup blueberry yogurt
- 1 banana, peeled, frozen
- 1/2 avocado, peeled, pitted
- 1 cup kale, stemmed, rinsed

DIRECTIONS

1. Gather all the ingredients.
2. Plug in a high-powered blender, and then add every one of the ingredients listed.
3. Turn it on for 45 to 60 seconds or extra dependent on the blender, until properly combined and smooth, and then divide the smoothie between two glasses.
4. Serve straight away.

Nutritions: *Calories: 441, Total Fat: 18g, Saturated Fat: 2g, Carbohydrates: 66g, Fiber: 10g, Sugars: 36g, Protein: 11g*

38. PINEAPPLE CELERY SMOOTHIE

PREPARATION: 5 MIN

COOKING: 0 MIN

SERVES: 1

INGREDIENTS

- 1/4 cup almond milk, unsweetened
- 1/2 pear, cored, chopped
- 1 stalk celery, chopped
- 1/2 banana, peeled, frozen
- 1/2 teaspoon honey
- 1/2 cup pineapple pieces, cubed

DIRECTIONS

1. Gather all the ingredients.
2. Plug in a high-powdered blender, and then add all the ingredients into it in the order mentioned in the list.
3. Turn it on for 45 to 60 seconds or more depending on the blender, until well blended and smooth, and then distribute the smoothie between two glasses.
4. Serve straight away.

Nutritions: *Calories: 205, Total Fat: 1.5g, Saturated Fat: 0.7g, Carbohydrates: 42.2g, Fiber: 5.7g, Sugars: 32.2g, Protein: 2.4g*

39. MANGO AND CUCUMBER SMOOTHIE

PREPARATION: 5 MIN

COOKING: 0 MIN

SERVES: 1

INGREDIENTS

- 1 ½ cup coconut milk, unsweetened
- 4 teaspoons lime juice
- 1 cup baby spinach leaves, fresh, rinsed
- 2 cup mango pieces, fresh or frozen
- 4 mint leaves, rinsed
- 1 cup chopped cucumber, deseeded, peeled
- 1/4 teaspoon cayenne pepper
- 1 cup ice cubes

DIRECTIONS

1. Collect all the ingredients.
2. Plug in a high-powered blender, along with all the ingredients into it in the directive mentioned in the list.
3. Pulse for 45 to 60 seconds or extra depending on the blender, up until well combined and smooth, and then distribute the smoothie between two glasses.
4. Serve straight away.

Nutritions: *Calories: 170, Total Fat: 4.6g, Saturated Fat: 0.5g, Carbohydrates: 33.5g, Fiber: 6g, Sugars: 28.2g, Protein: 2.6g*

40. MELON, KALE, AND BROCCOLI SMOOTHIE

PREPARATION: 5 MIN | COOKING: 0 MIN | SERVES: 1

INGREDIENTS

- 2 cups coconut water, unsweetened
- 2/3 cup broccoli florets
- 2 cups honeydew melon pieces
- 1 lime, peeled, deseeded, halved
- ½ cup kale, stemmed, rinsed
- 2 Medrol dates pitted
- ½ cup mint leaves
- 1 cup ice cubes

DIRECTIONS

1. Gather all the ingredients.
2. Plug in a high-powered blender, and then add all the ingredients in the order indicated in the list.
3. Pulse for 45 to 60 seconds or extra diverging on the blender, until well mixed and smooth out, and then distribute the smoothie between two glasses.
4. Serve straight away.

Nutritions: *Calories: 220, Total Fat: 1g, Saturated Fat: 0.6g, Carbohydrates: 46g, Fiber: 8.6g, Sugars: 39g, Protein: 5.4g*

41. AVOCADO AND CUCUMBER SMOOTHIE

PREPARATION: 5 MIN

COOKING: 0 MIN

SERVES: 1

INGREDIENTS

- 1 cup water, chilled
- 1 large cucumber, deseeded
- 1 avocado, cored, peeled

DIRECTIONS

1. Gather all the ingredients.
2. Plug in a high-powered blender, then combine all the ingredients into it in the order mentioned in the register.
3. Thump for 45 to 60 seconds or more dependent on the blender, until nicely combined and smooth, and then divide the smoothie between two glasses.
4. Serve straight away.

Nutritions: *Calories: 141, Total Fat: 9.8g, Saturated Fat: 1.5g, Carbohydrates: 10.2g, Fiber: 6.4g, Sugars: 2.7g, Protein: 1.7g*

42. APPLE, BANANA, AND COLLARD GREENS SMOOTHIE

PREPARATION: 5 MIN

COOKING: 0 MIN

SERVES: 1

INGREDIENTS

- 1 cup water, chilled
- 2 green apples, cored
- 1 large banana, peeled, frozen
- 1 ½ cup collard greens, frozen

DIRECTIONS

1. Gather all the ingredients.
2. Plug in a high powdered blender, and then combine the whole ingredients into it in the directive mentioned in the list.
3. Pulse for 45 to 60 seconds or more varying on the blender, until well blended and smooth, and then allocate the smoothie between two glasses.
4. Serve straight away.

Nutritions: *Calories: 179, Total Fat: 0.6g, Saturated Fat: 0.2g, Carbohydrates: 40g, Fiber: 7.7g, Sugars: 27.3g, Protein: 3.1g*

43. BROCCOLI AND ORANGE SMOOTHIE

PREPARATION: 5 MIN

COOKING: 0 MIN

SERVES: 1

INGREDIENTS

- 1 cup water, chilled
- 2 broccoli heads
- 1 orange, peeled

DIRECTIONS

1. Gather all the ingredients.
2. Plug in a high-powered blender, and later add every one of the ingredients into it in the order stated in the list.
3. Pulse for 45 to 60 seconds or more depending on the blender, until well combined and smooth, and then distribute the smoothie between two glasses.
4. Serve straight away.

Nutritions: *Calories: 241, Total Fat: 2.1g, Saturated Fat: 0.7g, Carbohydrates: 43.3g, Fiber: 17.4g, Sugars: 16.5g, Protein: 11.3g*

44. SWEET KIWI AND MINT SMOOTHIE

PREPARATION: 5 MIN

COOKING: 0 MIN

SERVES: 1

INGREDIENTS

- 1 cup water, chilled
- 2 kiwis, peeled
- 1 medium lemon, peeled
- ¼ cup mint leaves
- ¼ cup parsley leaves
- 2 teaspoons honey

DIRECTIONS

1. Gather all the ingredients.
2. Plug in a high-powered blender, and subsequently add all the ingredients into it in the order mentioned in the list.
3. Pulse for 45 to 60 seconds or extra differing on the blender, until perfectly combined and smooth out, and then divide the smoothie between two glasses.
4. Serve straight away.

Nutritions: *Calories: 81, Total Fat: 0.5g, Saturated Fat: 0.1g, Carbohydrates: 17.1g, Fiber: 3.4g, Sugars: 13g, Protein: 1.23g*

45. CUCUMBER, CELERY, AND APPLE SMOOTHIE

PREPARATION: 5 MIN

COOKING: 0 MIN

SERVES: 1

INGREDIENTS

- 1/2 cup water, chilled
- 1/4 lemon, juiced
- 1/2 large stalk of celery
- 1 medium green apple, cored
- 1/2 large cucumber

DIRECTIONS

1. Gather all the ingredients.
2. Plug in a high-powdered blender, and then add all the ingredients into it in the order indicated in the list.
3. Turn it on for 45 to 60 seconds or more differing on the blender, until properly combined and smooth, and then distribute the smoothie between two glasses.
4. Serve straight away.

Nutritions: *Calories: 131, Total Fat: 0.6g, Saturated Fat: 0.2g, Carbohydrates: 28.8g, Fiber: 6.7g, Sugars: 22.3g, Protein: 1.3g*

CHAPTER 8: SALADS

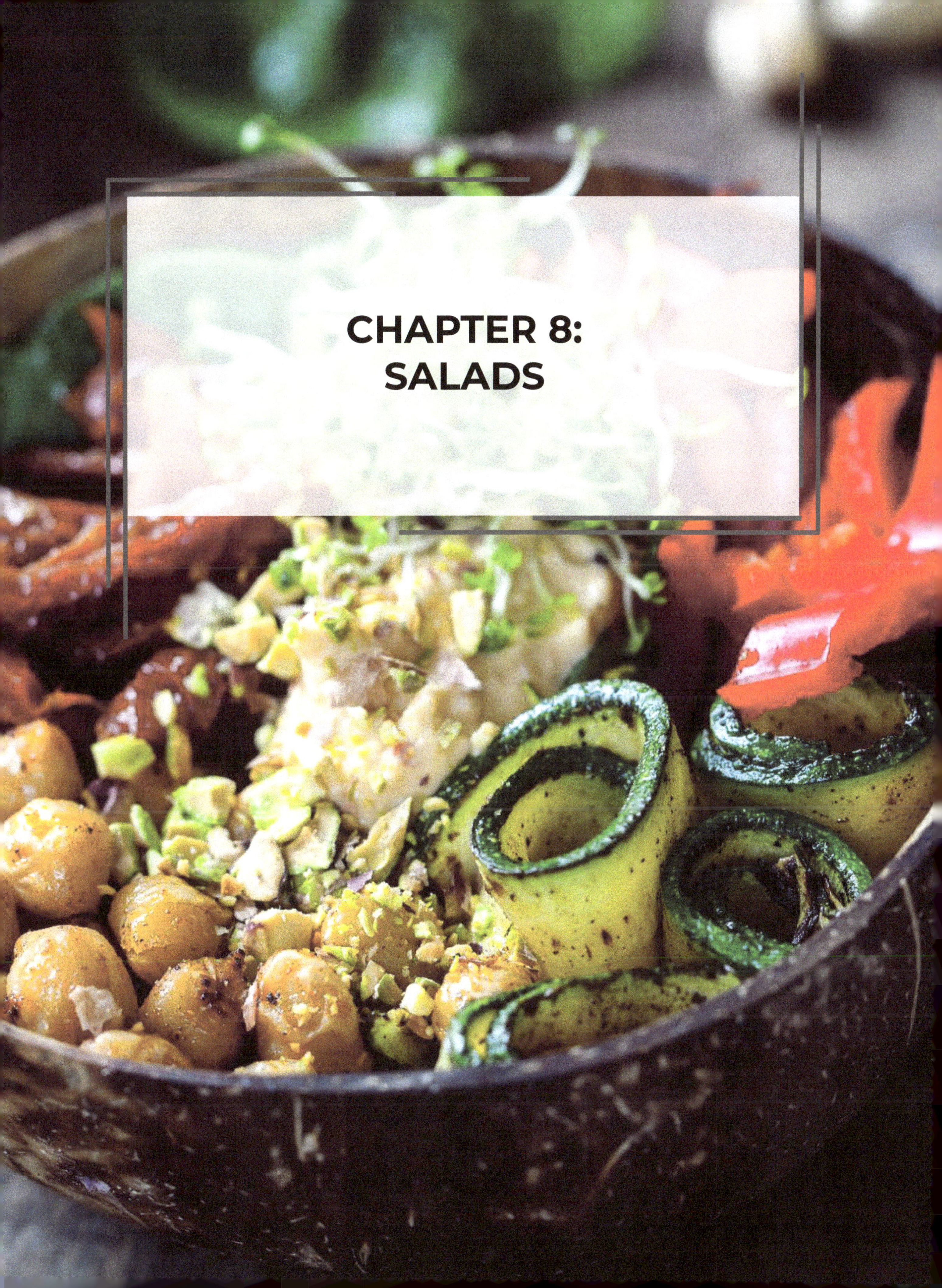

46. WASABI TUNA ASIAN SALAD

PREPARATION: 30 MIN

COOKING: 10 MIN

SERVES: 1

INGREDIENTS

- Lime juice (1 teaspoon)
- Non-stick cooking spray
- Pepper/dash of salt
- Wasabi paste (1 teaspoon)
- Olive oil (2 teaspoons)
- Chopped or shredded cucumbers (1/2 cup)
- Bok Choy stalks (1 cup)
- Raw tuna steak (8 oz.)

DIRECTIONS

1. Fish: preheat your skillet to medium heat. Mix your wasabi and lime juice; coat the tuna steaks.
2. Use a non-stick cooking spray on your skillet for 10 seconds.
3. Put your tuna steaks on the skillet and cook over medium heat until you get the desired doneness.
4. Salad: Slice the cucumber into match-stick tiny sizes. Cut the bok Choy into minute pieces. Toss gently with pepper, salt, and olive oil if you want.
5. Enjoy your food.

Nutritions: *Protein: 61g, Fiber: 1g, Cholesterol: 115mg, Saturated fats: 2g, Calories: 380*

47. LEMON GREEK SALAD

PREPARATION: 25 MIN

COOKING: 25 MIN

SERVES: 1

INGREDIENTS

- Chicken breast (140 oz)
- Chopped cucumber (1 cup)
- Chopped orange/red bell pepper (1 cup)
- Wedged/sliced/chopped tomatoes (1 cup)
- Chopped olives (1/4 cup)
- Fresh parsley (2 tablespoons), finely chopped.
- Finely chopped red onion (2 tablespoons)
- Lemon juice (5 teaspoons)
- Olive oil (1 teaspoon)
- Minced garlic (1 clove)

DIRECTIONS

1. Preheat your grill to medium heat.
2. Grill the chicken and cook on each side until the chicken is no longer pink or for 5 minutes.
3. Cut the chicken into tiny pieces. In your serving bowl, mix garlic, olives, and parsley. Whisk in olive oil (1 teaspoon) and lemon juice (4 teaspoons). Add onion, tomatoes, bell pepper, and cucumber.
4. Toss gently. Coat the ingredients with dressing. Add another teaspoon of lemon juice to taste. Divide the salad into two servings and put 6oz chicken on top of each salad.
5. Enjoy your meal.

Nutritions: *Protein: 56g, Fiber: 4g, Total carbs: 14g, Sodium: 280mg, Cholesterol: 145mg, Saturated fat: 2.5g, Total fat: 12g, Calories: 380*

48. BROCCOLI SALAD

PREPARATION: 5 MIN

COOKING: 25 MIN

SERVES: 1

INGREDIENTS

- 1/3 tablespoons sherry vinegar
- 1/24 cup olive oil
- 1/3 teaspoons fresh thyme, chopped
- 1/6 teaspoon Dijon mustard
- 1/6 teaspoon honey
- Salt to taste
- 1 1/3 cups broccoli florets
- 1/3 red onions
- 1/12 cup parmesan cheese shaved
- 1/24 cup pecans

DIRECTIONS

1. Mix the sherry vinegar, olive oil, thyme, mustard, honey, and salt in a bowl.
2. In a serving bowl, blend the broccoli florets and onions.
3. Drizzle the dressing on top.
4. Sprinkle with the pecans and parmesan cheese before serving.

Nutritions: *Calories: 199, Fat: 17.4g, Saturated fat: 2.9g, Carbohydrates: 7.5g, Fiber: 2.8g, Protein: 5.2g*

49. POTATO CARROT SALAD

PREPARATION: 15 MIN

COOKING: 10 MIN

SERVES: 1

INGREDIENTS

- Water
- 1 potato, sliced into cubes
- 1/2 carrots, cut into cubes
- 1/6 tablespoon milk
- 1/6 tablespoon Dijon mustard
- 1/24 cup mayonnaise
- Pepper to taste
- 1/3 teaspoons fresh thyme, chopped
- 1/6 stalk celery, chopped
- 1/6 scallions, chopped
- 1/6 slice turkey bacon, cooked crispy and crumbled

DIRECTIONS

1. Fill your pot with water.
2. Place it over medium-high heat.
3. Boil the potatoes and carrots for 10 to 12 minutes or until tender.
4. Drain and let cool.
5. In a bowl, mix the milk, mustard, mayonnaise, pepper, and thyme.
6. Stir in the potatoes, carrots, and celery.
7. Coat evenly with the sauce.
8. Cover and refrigerate for 4 hours.
9. Top with the scallions and turkey bacon bits before serving.

Nutritions: *Calories: 106, Fat: 5.3g, Saturated fat: 1g, Carbohydrates: 12.6g, Fiber: 1.8g, Protein: 2g*

50. MARINATED VEGGIE SALAD

PREPARATION: 4 H 30 MIN COOKING: 3 MIN SERVES: 1

INGREDIENTS

- 1 zucchini, sliced
- 4 tomatoes, sliced into wedges
- ¼ cup red onion, sliced thinly
- 1 green bell pepper, sliced
- 2 tablespoons fresh parsley, chopped
- 2 tablespoons red-wine vinegar
- 2 tablespoons olive oil
- 1 clove garlic, minced
- 1 teaspoon dried basil
- 2 tablespoons water
- Pine nuts, toasted and chopped

DIRECTIONS

1. In a bowl, combine the zucchini, tomatoes, red onion, green bell pepper, and parsley.
2. Pour the vinegar and oil into a glass jar with a lid.
3. Add the garlic, basil, and water.
4. Seal the jar and stir well to combine.
5. Pour the dressing into the vegetable mixture.
6. Cover the bowl.
7. Marinate in the refrigerator for 4 hours.
8. Garnish with the pine nuts before serving.

Nutritions: *Calories: 65, Fat: 4.7g, Saturated fat: 0.7g, Carbohydrates: 5.3g, Fiber: 1.2g, Protein: 0.9g*

51. MEDITERRANEAN SALAD

PREPARATION: 20 MIN

COOKING: 5 MIN

SERVES: 1

INGREDIENTS

- 1 teaspoon balsamic vinegar
- 1/2 tablespoon basil pesto
- 1/2 cup lettuce
- 1/8 cup broccoli florets, chopped
- 1/8 cup zucchini, chopped
- 1/8 cup tomato, chopped
- 1/8 cup yellow bell pepper, chopped
- 1/2 tablespoons feta cheese, crumbled

DIRECTIONS

1. Arrange the lettuce on a serving platter.
2. Top with the broccoli, zucchini, tomato, and bell pepper.
3. In a bowl, mix the vinegar and pesto.
4. Drizzle the dressing on top.
5. Sprinkle the feta cheese and serve.

Nutritions: *Calories: 100, Fat: 6g, Saturated fat: 1g, Carbohydrates: 7g, Protein: 4g*

52. POTATO TUNA SALAD

PREPARATION: 4 H 20 MIN COOKING: 10 MIN SERVES: 1

INGREDIENTS

- 1 potato, peeled and sliced into cubes
- 1/12 cup plain yogurt
- 1/12 cup mayonnaise
- 1/6 clove garlic, crushed and minced
- 1/6 tablespoon almond milk
- 1/6 tablespoon fresh dill, chopped
- ½ teaspoon lemon zest
- Salt to taste
- 1 cup cucumber, chopped
- ¼ cup scallions, chopped
- ¼ cup radishes, chopped
- (9 oz) canned tuna flakes
- 1/2 hard-boiled eggs, chopped
- 1 cups lettuce, chopped

DIRECTIONS

1. Fill your pot with water.
2. Add the potatoes and boil.
3. Cook for 15 minutes or till slightly tender.
4. Drain and let cool.
5. In a bowl, mix the yogurt, mayo, garlic, almond milk, fresh dill, lemon zest, and salt.
6. Stir in the potatoes, tuna flakes, and eggs.
7. Mix well.
8. Chill in the refrigerator for 4 hours.
9. Stir in the shredded lettuce before serving.

Nutritions: *Calories: 243, Fat: 9.9g, Saturated fat: 2g, Carbohydrates: 22.2g, Fiber: 4.6g, Protein: 17.5g*

53. HIGH PROTEIN SALAD

PREPARATION: 5 MIN

COOKING: 5 MIN

SERVES: 1

INGREDIENTS

Salad:

- 1(15 oz) can green kidney beans
- 1/4 tablespoon capers
- 1/4 handfuls arugula
- 1(15 oz) can lentils

Dressing:

- 1/1 tablespoon caper brine
- 1/1 tablespoon tamari
- 1/1 tablespoon balsamic vinegar
- 2/2 tablespoon peanut butter
- 2/2 tablespoon hot sauce
- 2/1 tablespoon tahini

DIRECTIONS

For the dressing:

1. In a bowl, stir all the ingredients until they come together to form a smooth dressing.

For the salad:

2. Mix the beans, arugula, capers, and lentils. Top with the dressing and serve.

Nutritions: *Calories: 205, Fat: 2g, Protein: 13g, Carbs: 31g, Fiber: 17g*

54. RICE AND VEGGIE BOWL

PREPARATION: 5 MIN

COOKING: 15 MIN

SERVES: 1

INGREDIENTS

- 1/3 tablespoon coconut oil
- 1/2 teaspoon ground cumin
- 1/2 teaspoon ground turmeric
- 1/3 teaspoon chili powder
- 1 red bell pepper, chopped
- 1/2 tablespoon tomato paste
- 1 bunch of broccoli, cut into bite-sized florets with short stems
- 1/2 teaspoon salt, to taste
- 1 large red onion, sliced
- 1/2 garlic cloves, minced
- 1/2 head of cauliflower, sliced into bite-sized florets
- 1/2 cups cooked rice
- Newly ground black pepper to taste

DIRECTIONS

1. Start with warming up the coconut oil over medium-high heat.
2. Stir in the turmeric, cumin, chili powder, salt, and tomato paste.
3. Cook the content for 1 minute. Stir repeatedly until the spices are fragrant.
4. Add the garlic and onion. Fry for 2 to 3 minutes until the onions are softened.
5. Add the broccoli, cauliflower, and bell pepper. Cover then cook for 3 to 4 minutes and stir occasionally.
6. Add the cooked rice. Stir so it will combine well with the vegetables. Cook for 2 to 3 minutes. Stir until the rice is warm.
7. Check the seasoning and change to taste if desired.
8. Lessen the heat and cook on low for 2 to 3 more minutes so the flavors will meld.
9. Serve with freshly ground black pepper.

Nutritions: *Calories: 260, Fat: 9g, Protein: 9g, Carbs: 36g, Fiber: 5g*

55. SQUASH BLACK BEAN BOWL

PREPARATION: 5 MIN

COOKING: 20 MIN

SERVES: 1

INGREDIENTS

- 1 large spaghetti squash, halved,
- 1/3 cup water (or 2 tablespoon olive oil, rubbed on the inside of squash)

Black bean filling:

- 1/2 (15 oz) can of black beans, emptied and rinsed
- 1/2 cup fire-roasted corn (or frozen sweet corn)
- 1/2 cup thinly sliced red cabbage
- 1/2 tablespoon chopped green onion, green and white parts
- ¼ cup chopped fresh coriander
- ½ lime, juiced or to taste
- Pepper and salt, to taste

Avocado mash:

- One ripe avocado, mashed
- ½ lime, juiced or to taste
- ¼ teaspoon cumin
- Pepper and pinch of sea salt

DIRECTIONS

1. Preheat the oven to 400°F.
2. Chop the squash in part and scoop out the seeds with a spoon, like a pumpkin.
3. Fill the roasting pan with 1/3 cup of water. Lay the squash, cut side down, in the pan. Bake for 30 minutes until soft and tender.
4. While this is baking, mix all the ingredients for the black bean filling in a medium-sized bowl.
5. In a small dish, crush the avocado and blend in the ingredients for the avocado mash.
6. Eliminate the squash from the oven and let it cool for 5 minutes. Scrape the squash with a fork so that it looks like spaghetti noodles. Then, fill it with black bean filling and top with avocado mash.
7. Serve and enjoy.

Nutritions: *Calories: 85, Fat: 0.5g, Protein: 4g, Carbs: 6g, Fiber: 4g*

56. PEA SALAD

PREPARATION: 40 MIN

COOKING: 0 MIN

SERVES: 1

INGREDIENTS

- 1/2 cup chickpeas, rinsed and drained
- 1/2 cups peas, divided
- Salt to taste
- 1 tablespoon olive oil
- ½ cup buttermilk
- Pepper to taste
- 2 cups pea greens
- 1/2 carrots shaved
- 1/4 cup snow peas, trimmed

DIRECTIONS

1. Add the chickpeas and half of the peas in your food processor.
2. Season with the salt.
3. Pulse until smooth. Set aside.
4. In a bowl, toss the remaining peas in oil, milk, salt, and pepper.
5. Transfer the mixture to your food processor.
6. Process until pureed.
7. Transfer this mixture to a bowl.
8. Arrange the pea greens on a serving plate.
9. Top with the shaved carrots and snow peas.
10. Stir in the pea and milk dressing.
11. Serve with the reserved chickpea hummus.

Nutritions: *Calories: 214, Fat: 8.6g, Saturated fat: 1.5g, Carbohydrates: 27.3g, Fiber: 8.4g, Protein: 8g*

57. SNAP PEA SALAD

PREPARATION: 1 H

COOKING: 0 MIN

SERVES: 1

INGREDIENTS

- 1/2 tablespoons mayonnaise
- ¾ teaspoon celery seed
- ¼ cup cider vinegar
- 1/2 teaspoon yellow mustard
- 1/2 tablespoon sugar
- Salt and pepper to taste
- 1 oz. radishes, sliced thinly
- 2 oz. sugar snap peas, sliced thinly

DIRECTIONS

1. In a bowl, combine the mayonnaise, celery seeds, vinegar, mustard, sugar, salt, and pepper.
2. Stir in the radishes and snap peas.
3. Refrigerate for 30 minutes.

Nutritions: *Calories: 69, Fat: 3.7g, Saturated fat: 0.6g, Carbohydrates: 7.1g, Fiber: 1.8g, Protein: 2g*

58. CUCUMBER TOMATO CHOPPED SALAD

PREPARATION: 15 MIN

COOKING: 0 MIN

SERVES: 1

INGREDIENTS

- 1/4 cup light mayonnaise
- 1/2 tablespoon lemon juice
- 1/2 tablespoon fresh dill, chopped
- 1/2 tablespoon chive, chopped
- 1/4 cup feta cheese, crumbled
- Salt and pepper to taste
- 1/2 red onion, chopped
- 1/2 cucumber, diced
- 1/2 radish, diced
- 1 tomato, diced
- Chives, chopped

DIRECTIONS

1. Combine the mayonnaise, lemon juice, fresh dill, chives, feta cheese, salt, and pepper in a bowl.
2. Mix well.
3. Stir in the onion, cucumber, radish, and tomatoes.
4. Coat evenly.
5. Garnish with the chopped chives.

Nutritions: *Calories: 187, Fat: 16.7g, Saturated fat: 4.1g, Carbohydrates: 6.7g, Fiber: 2g, Protein: 3.3g*

59. ZUCCHINI PASTA SALAD

PREPARATION: 4 MIN

COOKING: 0 MIN

SERVES: 1

INGREDIENTS

- 1 tablespoon olive oil
- 1/2 teaspoons dijon mustard
- 1/3 tablespoons red-wine vinegar
- 1/2 clove garlic, grated
- 2 tablespoons fresh oregano, chopped
- 1/2 shallot, chopped
- ¼ teaspoon red pepper flakes
- 4 oz. zucchini noodles
- ¼ cup Kalamata olives pitted
- 1 cups cherry tomato, sliced in half
- ¾ cup parmesan cheese shaved

DIRECTIONS

1. Mix the olive oil, Dijon mustard, red wine vinegar, garlic, oregano, shallot, and red pepper flakes in a bowl.
2. Stir in the zucchini noodles.
3. Sprinkle on top the olives, tomatoes, and parmesan cheese.

Nutritions: *Calories: 299, Fat: 24.7g, Saturated fat: 5.1g, Carbohydrates: 11.6g, Fiber: 2.8g, Protein: 7g*

60. EGG AVOCADO SALAD

PREPARATION: 10 MIN

COOKING: 0 MIN

SERVES: 1

INGREDIENTS

- 1/2 avocado
- 1 hard-boiled egg, peeled and chopped
- 1/4 tablespoon mayonnaise
- 1/4 tablespoons freshly squeezed lemon juice
- ¼ cup celery, chopped
- 1/2 tablespoons chives, chopped
- Salt and pepper to taste

DIRECTIONS

1. Add the avocado to a large bowl.
2. Mash the avocado using a fork.
3. Stir in the egg and mash the eggs.
4. Add the mayonnaise, lemon juice, celery, chives, salt, and pepper.
5. Chill in the refrigerator for at least 2o to 30 minutes before serving.

Nutritions: *Calories: 224, Fat: 18g, Saturated fat: 3.9g, Carbohydrates: 6.1g, Fiber: 3.6g, Protein: 10.6g*

CHAPTER 9:
FIRST COURSES AND SOUPS

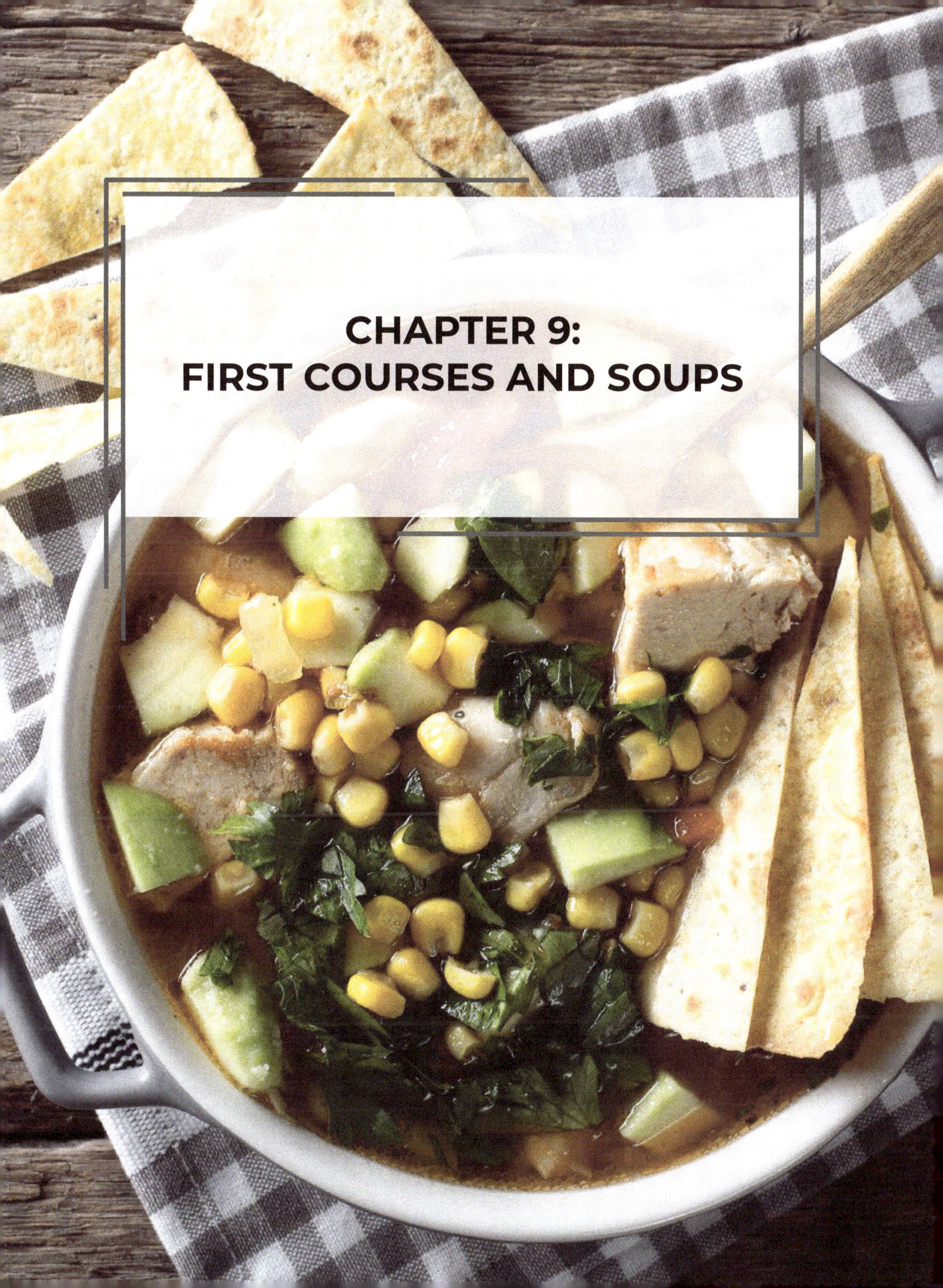

61. TOMATILLO AND GREEN CHILI PORK STEW

PREPARATION: 15 MIN

COOKING: 30 MIN

SERVES: 1

INGREDIENTS

- 1/2 scallions, chopped
- 1/2 cloves of garlic
- 1/4 pound tomatillos, trimmed and chopped
- 2 large romaine or green lettuce leaves, divided
- 1/2 serrano chilies, seeds, and membranes
- ½ teaspoon dried Mexican oregano (or you can use regular oregano)
- 1/4 pound of boneless pork loin, to be cut into bite-sized cubes
- ¼ cup coriander, chopped
- ¼ tablespoon (each) salt and paper
- 1/4 jalapeno, seeds, and membranes to be removed and thinly sliced
- 1/4 cup sliced radishes
- 1 lime wedge

DIRECTIONS

1. Combine scallions, garlic, tomatillos, four lettuce leaves, serrano chilies, and oregano in a blender. Then puree until smooth.
2. Put pork and tomatillo mixture in a medium pot. 1-inch of puree should cover the pork; if not, add water until it covers it. Season with pepper & salt, and cover it simmers. For 20 minutes, let it simmer on low heat.
3. Now, finely shred the remaining lettuce leaves.
4. When the stew is done cooking, garnish with coriander, radishes, finely shredded lettuce, sliced jalapenos, and lime wedges.

Nutritions: *Calories: 370, Protein: 36g, Carbohydrates: 14g, Fats: 19g*

62. OPTAVIA CLOUD BREAD

PREPARATION: 30 MIN

COOKING: 30 MIN

SERVES: 1

INGREDIENTS

- 1/4 cup fat-free 0%
- Plain Greek yogurt (4.4 oz)
- 1 egg, separated
- 1/32 teaspoon cream of tartar
- 1/2 packet sweetener (a granulated sweetener just like stevia)

DIRECTIONS

1. For about 30 minutes before making this meal, place the Kitchen Aid Bowl and the whisk attachment in the freezer.
2. Preheat your oven to 30 degrees.
3. Eliminate the bowl and whisk attachment from the freezer.
4. Separate the eggs. Now put the egg whites in the Kitchen Aid Bowl, and they should be in a different medium-sized bowl.
5. In the medium-sized bowl containing the yolks, mix in the sweetener and yogurt.
6. In the bowl containing the egg white, add in the cream of tartar. Beat this mixture until the egg whites turn to stiff peaks.
7. Now, take the egg yolk mixture and carefully fold it into the egg whites. Be cautious and avoid over-stirring.
8. On a parchment paper, place it then on a baking tray and spray with cooking spray.
9. Scoop out six equally sized "blobs" of the "dough" onto the parchment paper.

10. Bake for about 25–35 minutes (make sure you check when it is 25 minutes, in some ovens, they are done at this timestamp). You will know they are done as they will get brownish at the top and have some crack.
11. Most people like them cold against being warm.
12. Most people like to re-heat in a toast oven or toaster to get them a little bit crispy.

Nutritions: *Calories: 0, Protein: 0g, Carbohydrates: 0g, Fats: 0g*

63. ROSEMARY CAULIFLOWER ROLLS

PREPARATION: 15 MIN

COOKING: 20 MIN

SERVES: 1 (3 BISCUITS PER SERVING)

INGREDIENTS

- 1/12 cup almond flour
- 1 cup grated cauliflower
- 1/12 cup reduced-fat, shredded mozzarella, or cheddar cheese
- 1/2 eggs
- 1/2 tablespoons fresh rosemary, finely chopped
- ½ teaspoon salt

DIRECTIONS

1. Preheat your oven to 4000F.
2. Pour all the ingredients in a medium-sized bowl.
3. Scoop cauliflower mixture into 12 evenly sized rolls/biscuits onto a lightly greased and foil-lined baking sheet.
4. Bake until it turns golden brown, which should be achieved in about 30 minutes.
5. Note: if you want to have the outside of the rolls/biscuits crisp, then broil for some minutes before serving.

Nutritions: *Calories: 138, Protein: 11g, Carbohydrates: 8g, Fats: 7g*

64. TOMATO BRAISED CAULIFLOWER WITH CHICKEN

PREPARATION: 15 MIN

COOKING: 20 MIN

SERVES: 1

INGREDIENTS

- 1 garlic clove, sliced
- 3/4 scallions, to be trimmed and cut into 1-inch pieces
- 1/8 teaspoon dried oregano
- 1/8 teaspoon red pepper flakes
- 1/4 cups cauliflower
- 3/4 cups diced canned tomatoes
- 1/4 cup fresh basil, gently torn
- 1/8 teaspoon each of pepper and salt, divided
- 3/4 teaspoon olive oil
- 3/4 pound boneless, skinless chicken breasts

DIRECTIONS

1. Get a saucepan and combine the garlic, scallions, oregano, crushed red pepper, cauliflower, tomato, and add ¼ cup of water. Get everything boil together and add ¼ teaspoon of pepper and salt for seasoning, then cover the pot with a lid. Let it simmer for 10 minutes and stir as often as possible until you observe that the cauliflower is tender. Now, wrap up the seasoning with the remaining ¼ teaspoon of pepper and salt.
2. Using olive oil, toss the chicken breast and let it roast in the oven with the heat of 4500F for 20 minutes and an internal temperature of 1650F. Allow the chicken to rest for like 10 minutes.
3. Now slice the chicken and serve on a bed of tomato-braised cauliflower.

Nutritions: *Calories: 290, Fats: 10g, Carbohydrates: 13g, Protein: 38g*

65. CHEESEBURGER SOUP

PREPARATION: 15 MIN

COOKING: 30 MIN

SERVES: 1

INGREDIENTS

- 1/16 cup chopped onion
- 1 quantity of (14.5 oz) can dice tomato
- 1/4 pound 90% lean ground beef
- 3/16 cup chopped celery
- 1/4 teaspoons Worcestershire sauce
- 1/2 cup chicken broth
- 1/8 teaspoon salt
- 1/4 teaspoon dried parsley
- 2/3 cups of baby spinach
- 1/8 teaspoon ground pepper
- 1 oz. reduced-fat shredded cheddar cheese

DIRECTIONS

1. Get a large soup pot and cook the beef until it becomes brown. Add the celery, onion, and sauté until it becomes tender. Make sure to drain the excess liquid.
2. Stir in the broth, tomatoes, parsley, Worcestershire sauce, pepper, and salt. Cover and wait for it to simmer on low heat for about 20 minutes.
3. Add spinach and leave it to cook until it becomes wilted in about 1–3 minutes. Top each of your servings with 1 oz. of cheese.

Nutritions: *Calories: 400, Carbohydrates: 11g, Protein: 44g, Fats: 20g*

66. BRAISED COLLARD BEANS IN PEANUT SAUCE WITH PORK TENDERLOIN

PREPARATION: 25 MIN

COOKING:35 MIN

SERVES: 1

INGREDIENTS

- 1/2 cups chicken stock
- 3 cups chopped collard greens
- 1 1/2 tablespoons powdered peanut butter
- 3/4 cloves of garlic, crushed
- 1/4 teaspoon salt
- 1/8 teaspoon allspice
- 1/8 teaspoon black pepper
- 1/2 teaspoons lemon juice
- 3/8 teaspoon hot sauce
- 1/8 pound pork tenderloin

DIRECTIONS

1. Get a pot with a tight-fitting lid and combine the collards with the garlic, chicken stock, hot sauce, and half of the pepper and salt. Cook on low heat for about 1 hour or until the collards become tender.
2. Once the collards are tender, stir in the allspice, lemon juice. And they have powdered peanut butter. Keep warm.
3. Season the pork tenderloin with the remaining pepper and salt, and broil in a toaster oven for 10 minutes when you have an internal temperature of 1450F. Make sure to turn the tenderloin every 2 minutes to achieve an even browning all over. After that, you can take away the pork from the oven and allow it to rest for like 5 minutes.
4. Slice the pork as you will like and serve it on top of the braised greens.

Nutritions: *Calories: 320, Fats: 10g, Carbohydrates: 15g, Protein: 45g*

67. ZUCCHINI PIZZA CASSEROLE

PREPARATION: 15 MIN

COOKING: 50-60 MIN

SERVES: 1

INGREDIENTS

- ¼ teaspoon salt
- ¼ cup grated parmesan cheese
- 1/2 eggs
- 2/3 cups shredded unpeeled zucchini (this is about two medium zucchinis)
- 1 oz. reduced-fat, shredded cheddar cheese, divided
- 1 oz. reduced-fat, shredded mozzarella cheese, divided
- 1/8 pound 90–94% of lean ground beef
- Cooking spray
- 1 quantity 14.5 oz. can petite diced Italian tomatoes
- 1/8 cup chopped onion
- 1/2 small green bell pepper, chopped

DIRECTIONS

1. Preheat your oven to over 4000F.
2. Place zucchini in a strainer and sprinkle it with salt. Let it stand for about 10 minutes, and after that, press it to drain its moisture.
3. Combine zucchini with eggs, parmesan, and half of cheddar cheese and mozzarella.
4. Press the mixture into a lightly greased baking dish and bake while uncovered for about 20 minutes.
5. Cook the onion and beef in a medium skillet until it becomes done. Drain any leftover liquid and then stir in the tomatoes.
6. Pour the beef mixture over the zucchini and sprinkle with the remaining mozzarella cheese and cheddar. Top with green pepper
7. Bake for an extra 20 minutes or until it becomes heated all through.

Nutritions: *Calories: 478, Protein: 30g, Carbohydrates: 22g, Fats: 29g*

68. TOFU POWER BOWL

PREPARATION: 10 MIN

COOKING: 15-20 MIN

SERVES: 1

INGREDIENTS

- 15 oz. extra-firm tofu
- 1 teaspoon rice vinegar
- 2 tablespoons soy sauce
- 1 teaspoon sesame oil
- ½ cup grated cauliflower
- ½ cup grated eggplant
- ½ cup chopped kale

DIRECTIONS

1. Press tofu. Place tofu strips in multiple layers of paper towel or a clean dishcloth on top of a cutting board or plate. Place another of clean dish towels or paper towels on top of the tofu. Place a weight on top of this second layer (this can be a large plate with canned foods on top or hardcover books or a stack of leaves). Let it sit for not less than 15 minutes and then cut the tofu into 1-inch cubes.
2. Combine both the vinegar and soy sauce in a small bowl and whisk together.
3. Get a large skillet and heat the sesame oil in it. Place cubed tofu to cover one half of the skillet, and the cubed eggplant should cover the other half. Cook both together until they become slightly brown and tender in about 10–12 minutes. Remove from skillet and keep aside. Now, add kale and sauté until they become wilted in about 3–5 minutes.
4. Microwave the already grated cauliflower in a small bowl with one teaspoon of water for about 3–4 minutes until it becomes tender.
5. Arrange the cauliflower “rice” with tofu, eggplant, and kale in a bowl.

Nutritions: *Calories: 117, Protein: 14g, Carbohydrates: 2.2g, Fats: 7g*

69. GRILLED VEGGIE KABOBS

PREPARATION: 15 MIN

COOKING: 12-15 MIN

SERVES: 1

INGREDIENTS

Marinade:

- ½ cup balsamic vinegar
- 1/3 tablespoons minced thyme
- 1/4 tablespoons minced rosemary
- 1/2 cloves garlic, peeled and minced
- Sea salt, to taste (optional)
- Freshly ground black pepper, to taste

Veggies:

- 1/3 cups cherry tomatoes
- 1/3 red bell pepper, it should be seeded and cut into 1-inch pieces
- 1/3 green bell pepper, without seeds and cut into 1-inch pieces
- 1/3 medium yellow squash, cut into 1-inch rounds
- 1/3 medium zucchini, cut into 1-inch rounds
- 1/3 medium red onion skinned and cut into large chunks

Special Equipment:

- Two bamboo skewers, make sure to soak it in water for 30 minutes

DIRECTIONS

1. Preheat the grill to medium heat.
2. In making the marinade: In a small bowl, stir together the balsamic vinegar, thyme, rosemary, garlic, salt (if desired), and pepper.
3. Thread veggies onto skewers, alternating between different-colored veggies.
4. Grill the veggies for 12 to 15 minutes until softened and lightly charred, brushing the veggies with the marinade and flipping the skewers every 4 to 5 minutes.
5. Remove from the grill and serve hot.

Nutritions: *Calories: 98, Fat: 0.7g, Carbs: 19.2g, Protein: 3.8g, Fiber: 3.4g*

70. GRILLED CAULIFLOWER STEAKS

PREPARATION: 10 MIN | COOKING: 57 MIN | SERVES: 1

INGREDIENTS

- 1/2 medium heads cauliflower
- 1/2 medium shallots, peeled and minced
- Water, as needed
- 1/2 clove garlic, peeled and minced
- ½ teaspoon ground fennel
- ½ teaspoon minced sage
- ½ teaspoon crushed red pepper flakes
- ½ cup green lentils, rinsed
- 1/2 cups low-sodium vegetable broth
- Salt, to taste (optional)
- Freshly ground black pepper, to taste
- Chopped parsley, for garnish

DIRECTIONS

1. On a flat work surface, cut each of the cauliflower heads in half through the stem, then trim each half, so you get a 1-inch-thick steak.
2. Arrange each piece on a baking sheet and set aside. You can reserve the extra cauliflower florets for other uses.
3. Sauté the shallots in a medium saucepan over medium heat for 10 minutes, stirring occasionally. Add water, 1 to 3 tablespoons at a time, to keep the shallots from sticking.
4. Stir in the garlic, fennel, sage, red pepper flakes, and lentils and cook for 3 minutes.
5. Pour into the vegetable broth and bring to a boil over high heat.
6. Reduce the heat to medium, cover, and cook for 45 to 50 minutes, or until the lentils are very soft, adding more water as needed.
7. Using an immersion blender, purée the mixture until smooth. Sprinkle with salt (if desired) and pepper. Keep warm and set aside.
8. Preheat the grill to medium heat.
9. Grill the cauliflower steaks for about 7 minutes per side until evenly browned.
10. Transfer the cauliflower steaks to a plate and spoon the purée over them. Serve garnished with the parsley.

Nutritions: *Calories: 105, Fat: 1.1g, Carbs: 18.3g, Protein: 5.4g, Fiber: 4.9g*

71. VEGETABLE HASH WITH WHITE BEANS

PREPARATION: 15 MIN

COOKING: 23 MIN

SERVES: 1

INGREDIENTS

- 1 leek (white part only), finely chopped
- 1 red bell pepper, deseeded and diced
- Water, as needed
- 2 teaspoons minced rosemary
- 3 cloves garlic, peeled and minced
- 1 medium sweet potato, peeled and diced
- 1 enormous turnip, peeled and diced
- 2 cups cooked white beans, or 1 (15-oz./425-g) can drain and rinse
- Zest and juice of 1 orange
- 1 cup chopped kale
- Salt, to taste (optional)
- Freshly ground black pepper, to taste

DIRECTIONS

1. Put the leek and red pepper in a large saucepan over medium heat and sauté for 8 minutes, stir occasionally. Add water, 1 to 3 tablespoons at a time, to keep them from sticking to the bottom of the pan.
2. Stir in the rosemary and garlic and sauté for 1 minute more.
3. Add the sweet potato, turnip, beans, and orange juice and zest, and stir okay—heat until the vegetables are softened.
4. Add the kale and sprinkle with salt (if desired) and pepper. Cook for about 5 minutes or more until the kale is wilted.
5. Serve on a plate.

Nutritions: *Calories: 245, Fat: 0.6g, Carbs: 48.0g, Protein: 11.9g, Fiber: 9.3g*

72. RATATOUILLE

PREPARATION: 20 M

COOKING: 25 MIN

SERVES: 1

INGREDIENTS

- 1 medium red onion, peeled and diced
- Water, as needed
- 4 cloves garlic, peeled and minced
- 1 medium red bell pepper, without seeds and diced
- 1 small zucchini, diced
- 1 medium eggplant stemmed and diced
- 1 large tomato, diced
- ½ cup chopped basil
- Salt, to taste (optional)
- Freshly ground black pepper, to taste

DIRECTIONS

1. Put the onion in a medium saucepan over medium heat and sauté for 10 minutes, stirring occasionally, or until the onion is tender. Add water 1 to 3 tablespoons at a time to keep it from sticking.
2. Add the garlic, red pepper, zucchini, and eggplant and stir well. Lid the saucepan and cook for 12 to 15 minutes, stirring occasionally.
3. Mix in the tomatoes and basil, then sprinkle with salt (if desired) and pepper. Serve immediately.

Nutritions: *Calories: 76, Fat: 0.5g, Carbs: 15.3g, Protein: 2.7g, Fiber: 5.9g*

73. BAINGAN BHARTA (INDIAN SPICED EGGPLANT)

PREPARATION: 15 MIN

COOKING: 25 MIN

SERVES: 1

INGREDIENTS

- 1/2 medium onions, peeled and diced
- 1/4 medium red bell pepper, deseeded and diced
- Water, as needed
- 1/2 large tomatoes, finely chopped
- 1/2 medium eggplants, stemmed, peeled, and cut into ½-inch dices
- 3/4 tablespoons grated ginger
- 1/4 teaspoon coriander seed, toasted and ground
- 1/2 teaspoons cumin seeds, toasted and ground
- ½ teaspoon crushed red pepper flakes
- Pinch cloves
- Salt, to taste (optional)
- 1/2 coriander, leaves, and tender stems, finely sliced

DIRECTIONS

1. Combine the onions and red pepper in a large saucepan and cook over medium heat for about 10 to 12 minutes. Include water 1 to 2 tablespoons now to keep them from sticking to the pan.
2. Stir in the tomatoes, eggplant, ginger, coriander, cumin, crushed red pepper flakes, and cloves and cook for just about 12 to 15 minutes, or until the vegetables are tender.
3. Sprinkle with the salt, if desired. Garnish with the coriander and serve warm.

Nutritions: *Calories: 140, Fat: 1.1g, Carbs: 27.9g, Protein: 4.7g, Fiber: 10.9g*

74. KALE AND PINTO BEAN ENCHILADA CASSEROLE

PREPARATION: 10 MIN

COOKING: 30 MIN

SERVES: 1

INGREDIENTS

- 1/2 teaspoon olive oil (optional)
- 1/2 yellow onion, diced
- 1/2 bunch kale stemmed and chopped
- 1/4 teaspoons taco seasoning
- 1/2 to 2/3 cups cooked pinto beans, or 2 (15-oz./425-g) cans pinto beans, drained and rinsed
- Sea salt, to taste (optional)
- Black pepper, to taste
- 1/2 (16-oz./454-g) jar salsa (any variety), divided
- 2 corn tortillas
- ½ cup cashew cheese, or more to taste

DIRECTIONS

1. Preheat the oven to 350°F (205°C). Grease a baking dish with the olive oil, if desired.
2. Place the onion, kale, taco seasoning, and beans in the dish. Then sprinkle with salt (if desired) and pepper. Drizzle half the salsa over the beans. Next, place the tortillas on top. Scatter with the remaining salsa and cashew cheese.
3. Before baking, cover the dish with an aluminum foil in the preheated oven for about 30 minutes or until the vegetables are warm and the salsa bubbles.
4. Let it cool for 10 minutes before slicing and serving.

Nutritions: *Calories: 194, Fat: 3.8g, Carbs: 29.0g, Protein: 10.9g, Fiber: 9.4g*

75. POTATO AND ZUCCHINI CASSEROLE

PREPARATION: 10 MIN

COOKING: 1 H

SERVES: 1

INGREDIENTS

- 1/2 large russet potatoes halved lengthwise and thinly sliced
- 1/2 medium zucchinis halved lengthwise and thinly sliced
- 1/4 cup nutritional yeast
- 1/4 cup diced green or red bell pepper (about one small bell pepper)
- 1/4 cup diced red, white, or yellow onion (about one small onion)
- 1/8 cup dry breadcrumbs
- 1/8 cup olive oil (optional)
- 2/3 teaspoons minced garlic (about three small cloves)
- Pepper, to taste
- Sea salt, to taste (optional)

DIRECTIONS

1. Preheat the oven to 400°F.
2. Mix all the ingredients.
3. Place the mixture in a large cooking pot dish.
4. Bake in the preheated oven for 1 hour until heated through, stirring once halfway through.
5. Take out of the oven and allow to cool for 5 minutes before serving.

Nutritions: *Calories: 352, Fat: 10.0g, Carbs: 51.5g, Protein: 14.1g, Fiber: 5.5g*

76. BROCCOLI CASSEROLE WITH BEANS AND WALNUTS

PREPARATION: 10 MIN

COOKING: 35-40 MIN

SERVES: 1

INGREDIENTS

- 1/4 cup vegetable broth
- 1/2 broccoli heads, crowns, and stalks finely chopped
- 1/3 teaspoon salt (optional)
- 2/5 cups cooked pinto or navy beans
- 1/2 to 2/3 tablespoons brown rice flour or arrowroot flour
- 1/4 cup chopped walnuts

DIRECTIONS

1. Preheat the oven to 400°F (205°C).
2. Warm the vegetable broth in a large ovenproof pot over medium heat.
3. Add the broccoli and season with salt, if desired, then cook for 6 to 8 minutes, stirring occasionally, or until the broccoli is light green.
4. Add the pinto beans and brown rice flour to the skillet and stir well. Sauté for another 5 to 7 minutes, or until the liquid thickens slightly. Scatter the top with the walnuts.
5. Transfer the pot to the oven. Bake it until the walnuts are toasted, 20 to 25 minutes.
6. Let the casserole cool for 8 to 10 minutes in the pot before serving.

Nutritions: *Calories: 412, Fat: 20.2g, Carbs: 43.3g, Protein: 21.6g, Fiber: 13.1g*

77. PISTACHIO CRUSTED TOFU

PREPARATION: 10 MIN

COOKING: 20 MIN

SERVES: 1

INGREDIENTS

- 1/8 cup roasted, shelled pistachios
- 1/8 cup whole-wheat breadcrumbs
- 1/4 garlic clove, minced
- 1/4 shallot, minced
- 1/8 teaspoon dried tarragon
- 1/4 teaspoon grated lemon zest
- Sea salt, to taste (optional)
- Black pepper, to taste
- 1/4 (16-oz./454-g) package sprouted or extra-firm tofu, drained and sliced lengthwise into eight pieces
- 1/8 tablespoon dijon mustard
- 1/8 tablespoon lemon juice

DIRECTIONS

1. Warm up the oven to 400°F (205°C). Line a baking sheet with parchment paper.
2. Then place the pistachios in a food processor until they are about the size of the breadcrumbs. Mix the pistachios, breadcrumbs, garlic, shallot, tarragon, and lemon zest in a shallow dish. Sprinkle with salt (if desired) and pepper. Set aside.
3. Sprinkle the tofu with salt (if desired) and pepper. Mix the mustard and lemon juice in a small bowl and stir well.
4. Brush all over the tofu with the mustard mixture, then coat each slice with the pistachio mixture.
5. Arrange the tofu on the baking sheet. Scatter any remaining pistachio mixture over the slices.
6. Bake in the warmed oven for about 18 to 20 minutes, or until the tofu is browned and crispy.
7. Serve hot.

Nutritions: *Calories: 159, Fat: 9.3g, Carbs: 8.3g, Protein: 10.4g, Fiber: 1.6g*

78. AIR FRYER ASPARAGUS

PREPARATION: 5 MIN

COOKING: 8 MIN

SERVES: 1

INGREDIENTS

- Nutritional yeast
- Olive oil non-stick spray
- 1 bunch of asparagus

DIRECTIONS

1. Prepare the ingredients. Wash asparagus. Do not forget to trim off thick, woody ends.
2. Spray asparagus with olive oil spray and sprinkle with yeast.
3. Air Frying. In your Instant Crisp Air Fryer, lay asparagus in a singular layer. Set the temperature to 360°F. While the time limit to 8 minutes.

Nutritions: *Calories: 17, Fat: 4g, Protein: 9g*

79. AVOCADO FRIES

PREPARATION: 10 MIN | COOKING: 7 MIN | SERVES: 1

INGREDIENTS

- 1 avocado
- 1/8 teaspoon salt
- 1/4 cup panko breadcrumbs
- Bean liquid (Aquafaba) from a 15-oz. can of white or garbanzo beans

DIRECTIONS

1. Prepare the ingredients. Peel, pit, and slice up avocado.
2. Toss salt and breadcrumbs together in a bowl. Place Aquafaba into another bowl.
3. Dredge slices of avocado first in Aquafaba and then in panko, making sure you can even coating.
4. Air Frying. Place coated avocado slices into a single layer in the Instant Crisp Air Fryer. Set temperature to 390°F and set time to 5 minutes.
5. Serve with your favorite Keto dipping sauce!

Nutritions: *Calories: 102, Fat: 22g, Protein: 9g, Sugar: 1g*

80. BELL-PEPPER CORN WRAPPED IN TORTILLA

PREPARATION: 5 MIN

COOKING: 15 MIN

SERVES: 1

INGREDIENTS

- 1/4 small red bell pepper, chopped
- 1/4 small yellow onion, diced
- 1/4 tablespoon water
- 1/2 cobs grilled corn kernels
- 1 large tortilla
- 1 piece commercial vegan nuggets, chopped
- Mixed greens for garnish

DIRECTIONS

1. Prepare the ingredients. Preheat the Instant Crisp Air Fryer to 400°F.
2. In a skillet heated over medium heat, water sautés the vegan nuggets and the onions, bell peppers, and corn kernels. Set aside.
3. Place filling inside the corn tortillas.
4. Air Frying. Lock the air fryer lid. Fold the tortillas and place inside the Instant Crisp Air Fryer and cook for 15 minutes until the tortilla wraps are crispy.
5. Serve with mixed greens on top.

Nutritions: *Calories: 548, Fat: 20.7g, Protein: 46g*

81. CAULIFLOWER RICE

PREPARATION: 5 MIN

COOKING: 20 MIN

SERVES: 1

INGREDIENTS

Round 1:

- 1/2 teaspoon turmeric
- 1/2 cup diced carrot
- 1/8 cup diced onion
- 1/2 tablespoon low-sodium soy sauce
- 1/8 block extra firm tofu

Round 2:

- ½ cup frozen peas
- 1/4 minced garlic cloves
- ½ cup chopped broccoli
- 1/2 tablespoon minced ginger
- 1/4 tablespoon rice vinegar
- 1/4 teaspoon toasted sesame oil
- 1/2 tablespoon reduced-sodium soy sauce
- 1/2 cup riced cauliflower

DIRECTIONS

1. Prepare the ingredients. Crush tofu in a large bowl and toss with all the round one ingredient.
2. Air Frying. Lock the air fryer lid. Preheat the Instant Crisp Air Fryer to 370 degrees. Also, set the temperature to 370°F, set time to 10 minutes, and cook 10 minutes, making sure to shake once.
3. In another bowl, toss ingredients from round 2 together.
4. Add round 2 mixture to Instant Crisp Air Fryer and cook another 10 minutes to shake 5 minutes.
5. Enjoy!

Nutritions: *Calories: 67, Fat: 8g, Protein: 3g, Sugar: 0g*

82. STUFFED MUSHROOMS

PREPARATION: 7 MIN

COOKING: 8 MIN

SERVES: 1

INGREDIENTS

- 1/2 rashers bacon, diced
- ½ onion, diced
- ½ bell pepper, diced
- 1/2 small carrot, diced
- 2 medium-size mushrooms (Separate the caps & stalks)
- 1/4 cup shredded cheddar plus extra for the top
- 1/4 cup sour cream

DIRECTIONS

1. Prepare the ingredients. Chop the mushrooms stalks finely and fry them up with the bacon, onion, pepper, and carrot at 350F° for 8 minutes.
2. Also, check when the veggies are tender, stir in the sour cream & the cheese. Keep on the heat until the cheese has melted, and everything is mixed nicely.
3. Now grab the mushroom caps and heap a plop of filling on each one.
4. Place in the fryer basket and top with a little extra cheese.

Nutritions: *Calories: 285, Fat: 20.5g, Protein: 8.6g*

83. ZUCCHINI OMELET

PREPARATION: 10 MIN

COOKING: 10 MIN

SERVES: 1

INGREDIENTS

- 1/2 teaspoon butter
- 1/2 zucchini, julienned
- 1 egg
- 1/8 teaspoon fresh basil, chopped
- 1/8 teaspoon red pepper flakes, crushed
- Salted and newly ground black pepper, to taste

DIRECTIONS

1. Prepare the ingredients. Preheat the Instant Crisp Air Fryer to 355°F.
2. Melt butter on a medium heat using a skillet.
3. Add zucchini and cook for about 3–4 minutes.
4. In a bowl, add the eggs, basil, red pepper flakes, salt, and black pepper and beat well.
5. Add cooked zucchini and gently stir to combine.
6. Air Frying. Transfer the mixture into the Instant Crisp Air Fryer pan. Lock the air fryer lid.
7. Cook for about 10 minutes. Also, you may opt to wait until it is done thoroughly.

Nutritions: *Calories: 285, Fat: 20.5g, Protein: 8.6g*

84. CHEESY CAULIFLOWER FRITTERS

PREPARATION: 10 MIN

COOKING: 7 MIN

SERVES: 1

INGREDIENTS

- ½ cup chopped parsley
- 1 cup Italian breadcrumbs
- 1/3 cup shredded mozzarella cheese
- 1/3 cup shredded sharp cheddar cheese
- 1 egg
- 2 minced garlic cloves
- 3 chopped scallions
- 1 head of cauliflower

DIRECTIONS

1. Prepare the ingredients. Cut the cauliflower up into florets. Wash well and pat dry. Place into a food processor and pulse 20–30 seconds until it looks like rice.
2. Place the cauliflower rice in a bowl and mix with pepper, salt, egg, cheeses, breadcrumbs, garlic, and scallions.
3. With hands, form 15 patties of the mixture then add more breadcrumbs if needed.
4. Air Frying. With olive oil, spritz patties, and put the fitters into your Instant Crisp Air Fryer. Pile it in a single layer. Lock the air fryer lid. Set temperature to 390°F, and set time to 7 minutes, flipping after 7 minutes.

Nutritions: *Calories: 209, Fat: 17g, Protein: 6g, Sugar: 0.5*

85. ZUCCHINI PARMESAN CHIPS

PREPARATION: 10 MIN

COOKING: 8 MIN

SERVES: 1

INGREDIENTS

- ½ teaspoon paprika
- ½ cup grated parmesan cheese
- ½ cup Italian breadcrumbs
- 1 lightly beaten egg
- 2 thinly sliced zucchinis

DIRECTIONS

1. Prepare the ingredients. Use a very sharp knife or mandolin slicer to slice zucchini as thinly as you can. Pat off extra moisture.
2. Beat egg with a pinch of pepper and salt and a bit of water.
3. Combine paprika, cheese, and breadcrumbs in a bowl.
4. Dip slices of zucchini into the egg mixture and then into breadcrumb mixture. Press gently to coat.
5. Air Frying. With olive oil cooking spray, mist encrusted zucchini slices. Put into your Instant Crisp Air Fryer in a single layer. Latch the air fryer lid. Set temperature to 350°F and set time to 8 minutes.
6. Sprinkle with salt and serve with salsa.

Nutritions: *Calories: 211, Fat: 16g, Protein: 8g, Sugar: 0g*

86. JALAPENO CHEESE BALLS

PREPARATION: 10 MIN

COOKING: 8 MIN

SERVES: 1

INGREDIENTS

- 1-oz. cream cheese
- 1/6 cup shredded mozzarella cheese
- 1/6 cup shredded cheddar cheese
- 1/2 jalapeños, finely chopped
- ½ cup breadcrumbs
- 2 eggs
- ½ cup all-purpose flour
- Salt
- Pepper
- Cooking oil

DIRECTIONS

1. Prepare the ingredients. Combine the cream cheese, mozzarella, cheddar, and jalapeños in a medium bowl. Mix well.
2. Form the cheese mixture into balls about an inch thick. You may also use a small ice cream scoop. It works well.
3. Arrange the cheese balls on a sheet pan and place in the freezer for 15 minutes. It will help the cheese balls maintain their shape while frying.
4. Spray the Instant Crisp Air Fryer basket with cooking oil. Place the breadcrumbs in a small bowl. In another small bowl, beat the eggs. In the third small bowl, combine the flour with salt and pepper to taste, and mix well. Remove the cheese balls from the freezer. Plunge the cheese balls in the flour, then the eggs, and the breadcrumbs.
5. Air Frying. Place the cheese balls in the Instant Crisp Air Fryer. Spray with cooking oil. Lock the air fryer lid. Cook for 8 minutes.
6. Open the Instant Crisp Air Fryer and flip the cheese balls. I recommend flipping them instead of shaking, so the balls maintain their form. Cook an additional 4 minutes. Cool before serving.

Nutritions: *Calories: 96, Fat: 6g, Protein: 4g, Sugar: 0g*

87. CRISPY ROASTED BROCCOLI

PREPARATION: 10 MIN

COOKING: 8 MIN

SERVES: 1

INGREDIENTS

- ¼ teaspoon masala
- ½ teaspoon red chili powder
- ½ teaspoon salt
- ¼ teaspoon turmeric powder
- 1 tablespoon chickpea flour
- 1 tablespoon yogurt
- ½ pound broccoli

DIRECTIONS

1. Prepare the ingredients. Cut broccoli up into florets. Immerse in a bowl of water with two teaspoons of salt for at least half an hour to remove impurities.
2. Take out broccoli florets from water and let drain. Wipe down thoroughly.
3. Mix all other ingredients to create a marinade.
4. Toss broccoli florets in the marinade. Cover and chill 15–30 minutes.
5. Air Frying. Preheat the Instant Crisp Air Fryer to 390 degrees. Place marinated broccoli florets into the fryer, lock the air fryer lid, set the temperature to 350°F, and set time to 10 minutes. Florets will be crispy when done.

Nutritions: *Calories: 96, Fat: 1.3g, Protein: 7g, Sugar: 4.5g*

88. COCONUT BATTERED CAULIFLOWER BITES

PREPARATION: 5 MIN

COOKING: 20 MIN

SERVES: 1

INGREDIENTS

- Salt and pepper to taste
- 1 flax egg or one tablespoon flaxseed meal + 3 tablespoon water
- 1 small cauliflower, cut into florets
- 1 teaspoon mixed spice
- ½ teaspoon mustard powder
- 2 tablespoons maple syrup
- 1 clove of garlic, minced
- 2 tablespoons soy sauce
- 1/3 cup oats flour
- 1/3 cup plain flour
- 1/3 cup desiccated coconut

DIRECTIONS

1. Prepare the ingredients.
2. In a mixing bowl, mix oats, flour, and desiccated coconut. Season with salt and pepper to taste. Set aside.
3. In another bowl, place the flax egg and add a pinch of salt to taste. Set aside.
4. Season the cauliflower with mixed spice and mustard powder.
5. Dredge the florets in the flax egg first, then in the flour mixture.
6. Air Frying. Place inside the Instant Crisp Air Fryer lock the air fryer lid and cook at 400°F or 15 minutes.
7. Meanwhile, place the maple syrup, garlic, and soy sauce in a saucepan and heat over medium flame. Wait for it to boil and adjust the heat to low until the sauce thickens.
8. After 15 minutes, take out the florets from the Instant Crisp Air Fryer and place them in the saucepan.
9. Toss to coat the florets and place inside the Instant Crisp Air Fryer and cook for another 5 minutes.

Nutritions: *Calories: 154, Fat: 2.3g, Protein: 4.69g*

89. CRISPY JALAPENO COINS

PREPARATION: 10 MIN | COOKING: 5 MIN | SERVES: 1

INGREDIENTS

- 1 egg
- 2–3 tablespoon coconut flour
- 1 sliced and seeded jalapeno
- Pinch garlic powder
- Pinch onion powder
- Bit cajun seasoning (optional)
- Pinch pepper and salt

DIRECTIONS

1. Prepare the ingredients. Ensure your Instant Crisp Air Fryer is preheated to 400 degrees.
2. Mix all dry ingredients.
3. Pat jalapeno slices dry. Dip coins into the egg wash and then into the dry mixture. Toss to coat thoroughly.
4. Add coated jalapeno slices to Instant Crisp Air Fryer in a singular layer. Spray with olive oil.
5. Air Frying. Lock the air fryer lid. Set temperature to 350°F and set time to 5 minutes. Cook just till crispy.

Nutritions: *Calories: 128, Fat: 8g, Protein: 7g, Sugar: 0g*

90. BUFFALO CAULIFLOWER

PREPARATION: 5 MIN COOKING: 15 MIN SERVES: 1

INGREDIENTS

Cauliflower:

- 1 cup panko breadcrumbs
- 1 teaspoon salt
- 2 cup cauliflower florets

Buffalo Coating:

- ¼ cup vegan buffalo sauce
- ¼ cup melted vegan butter

DIRECTIONS

1. Prepare the ingredients. Melt butter in microwave and whisk in buffalo sauce.
2. Dip each cauliflower floret into buffalo mixture, ensuring it gets coated well. Holdover a bowl till floret is done dripping.
3. Mix breadcrumbs with salt.
4. Air Frying. Dredge dipped florets into breadcrumbs and place them into Instant Crisp Air Fryer. Lock the air fryer lid. Set temperature to 350°F and set time to 15 minutes. When slightly browned, they are ready to eat!
5. Serve with your favorite Keto dipping sauce!

Nutritions: *Calories: 194, Fat: 17g, Protein: 10g, Sugar: 3*

CHAPTER 10: MEAT AND FISH DISHES

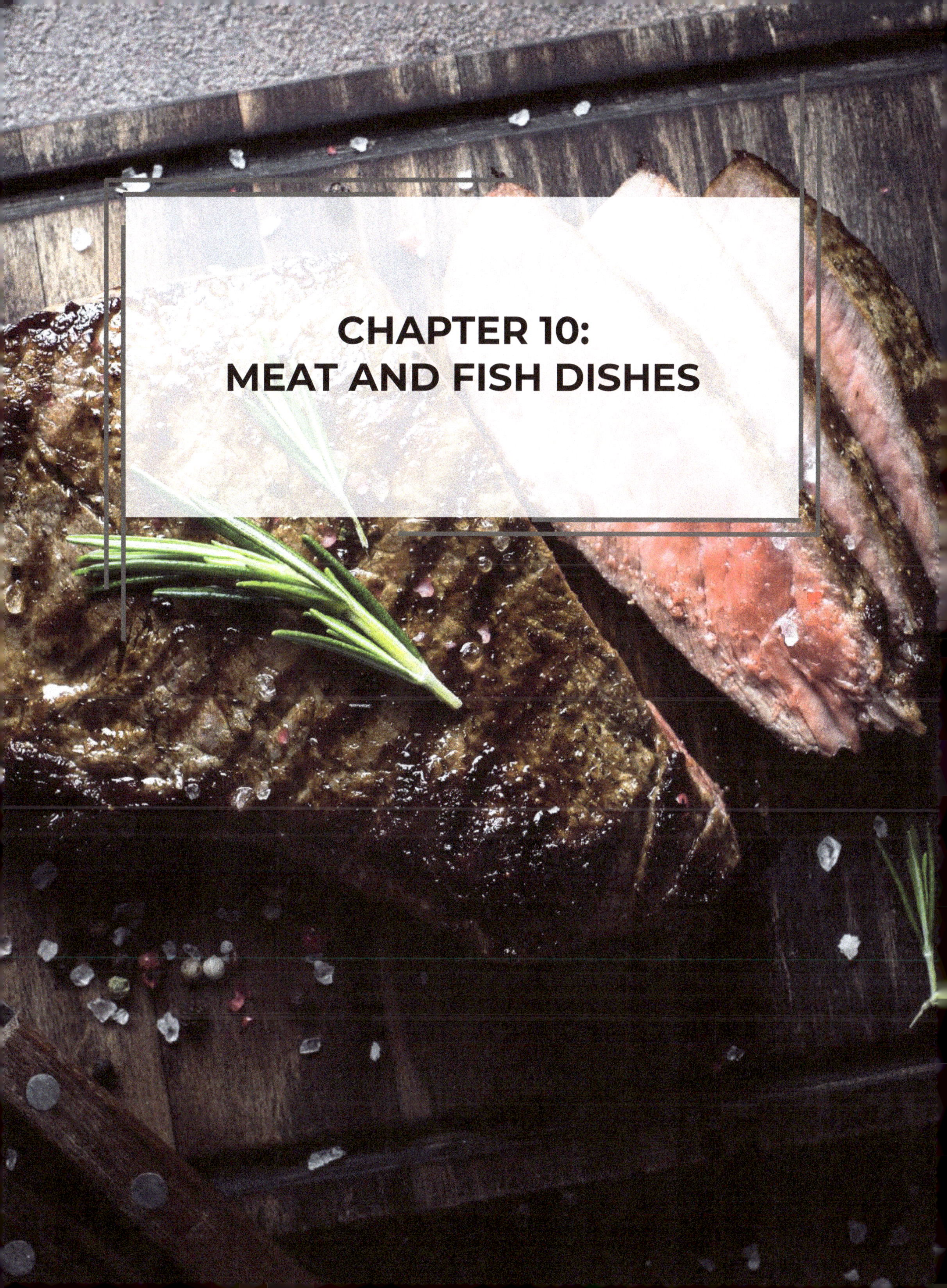

91. ASPARAGUS AND CRABMEAT FRITTATA

PREPARATION: 10-15 MIN   COOKING: 10-20 MIN   SERVES: 1

INGREDIENTS

- 1½ tablespoon extra-virgin olive oil
- 1 pound asparagus
- 1/2 teaspoon salt
- 1 ½ teaspoon black pepper
- 1/2 teaspoon sweet paprika
- 1/2 pound lump crabmeat
- 1/2 tablespoon finely cut chives
- ¼ cup basil chopped
- 1/2 cups liquid egg substitute

DIRECTIONS

1. Deter the tough ends of the asparagus and cut it into bite-sized pieces.
2. Preheat an oven to 375°F.
3. In a 12-Inch to a 14-inch oven-proof, non-stick skillet, warm the olive oil and sweat the asparagus until tender—season with pepper, paprika, and salt.
4. In a mixing bowl, add the chives, crabmeat, and basil.
5. Pour in the liquid egg substitute and mix until combined.
6. With the cooked asparagus, pour the crab and egg mixture into the skillet then stir to combine. Bake over low to medium heat until the eggs start bubbling.
7. Place the skillet inside the oven. Then, bake for about 15–20 minutes. Wait until the eggs are golden brown. Serve the dish warm.

Nutritions: *Calories: 340, Protein: 50g, Carbohydrates: 14g, Fats: 10g*

92. GRILLED CHICKEN POWER BOWL WITH GREEN GODDESS DRESSING

PREPARATION: 30 MIN

COOKING: 15 MIN

SERVES: 1

INGREDIENTS

- 1/3 boneless, skinless chicken breasts
- 1/8 teaspoon each salt & pepper
- 1/4 cup rice or cubed kabocha squash
- 1/4 cup diced zucchini
- 1/4 cup rice yellow summer squash
- 1/4 cup rice broccoli
- 2 cherry tomatoes halved
- 1 radish, sliced thin
- 1/4 cup shredded red cabbage
- 1/8 cup hemp or pumpkin seeds
- Green goddess dressing
- ½ cup low-fat plain Greek yogurt
- 1/4 cup fresh basil
- 1/4 clove garlic
- 1 tablespoon lemon juice
- ¼ teaspoon each salt & pepper

DIRECTIONS

1. Preheat oven to 350°F.
2. Season chicken with salt and pepper.
3. Roast chicken about 10–12 minutes or until it reaches a temperature of 165°F. When done, dismiss from oven and set aside to rest about 5 minutes. Cut into bite-sized pieces and keep warm.
4. While the chicken rests, steam riced kabocha squash, yellow summer squash, zucchini, and broccoli in a covered microwave-proof bowl about 5 minutes till tender.
5. For the dressing, arrange the ingredients in a blender and puree till smooth.
6. To serve into four individual serving bowls, put an equal amount of the riced veggie mixture. Make sure to add an equal amount of cherry tomatoes, radishes, and shredded cabbage to each bowl. Also, each bowl should contain a quarter of the chicken and one tablespoon of seeds—drizzle dressing on top. Enjoy!

Nutritions: *Calories: 300, Protein: 43g, Carbohydrates: 12g, Fats: 10g*

93. BACON CHEESEBURGER

PREPARATION: 5 MIN

COOKING: 15 MIN

SERVES: 1

INGREDIENTS

- 1/4 pound lean ground beef
- ¼ cup chopped yellow onion
- 1/4 clove garlic, minced
- 1/4 tablespoon yellow mustard
- 1/4 tablespoon Worcestershire sauce
- 1/8 teaspoon salt
- Cooking spray
- 1 ultra-thin slice cheddar cheese, cut into six equal-sized rectangular pieces
- 1piece of turkey bacon, each cut into eight evenly sized rectangular pieces
- 3 dill pickle chips
- 1–2 green leaf lettuce leaves, torn into 24 small square-shaped pieces
- 2 cherry tomatoes, sliced in half

DIRECTIONS

1. Preheat oven to 400°F.
2. Combine the garlic, salt, onion, Worcestershire sauce, and beef in a medium-sized bowl, and mix well.
3. Form mixture into 24 small meatballs. Put meatballs onto a foil-lined baking sheet and cook for 12–15 minutes. Leave oven.
4. Top every meatball with a piece of cheese, then go back to the oven till cheese melts, about 2 to 3 minutes. Let meatballs cool.
5. To assemble bites: on a toothpick layer, a cheese-covered meatball, piece of bacon, piece of lettuce, pickle chip, and a tomato half.

Nutritions: *Calories: 303, Protein: 15g, Carbohydrates: 30g, Fats: 14g*

94. ANCHO TILAPIA ON CAULIFLOWER RICE

PREPARATION: 10 MIN COOKING: 20 MIN SERVES: 1

INGREDIENTS

- 1/2 lbs. tilapia
- 1/4 teaspoon lime juice
- 1/4 teaspoon salt
- 1/4 tablespoon ground ancho pepper
- 1/4 teaspoon ground cumin
- 3/4 tablespoon extra-virgin olive oil
- 1/16 cup toasted pumpkin seeds
- 3/2 cups cauliflower rice minutes
- 1/4 cup coarsely chopped fresh coriander

DIRECTIONS

1. Preheat oven to 450°F.
2. Dress tilapia with lime juice and set aside.
3. Combine cumin, ancho pepper, and salt in a bowl—season tilapia with spice mixture.
4. Lay tilapia on a baking sheet or casserole dish and bake for 7 minutes.
5. In the meantime, in a big skillet, sweat the cauliflower rice in olive oil till tender, about 2–3 minutes.
6. Blend the pumpkin seeds and coriander into the rice. Dismiss from heat and serve.

Nutritions: *Calories: 350, Protein: 51g, Carbohydrates: 10g, Fats: 10g*

95. TURKEY CAPRESE MEATLOAF CUPS

PREPARATION: 10 MIN

COOKING: 35 MIN

SERVES: 1

INGREDIENTS

- 1/4 large egg
- 1/4 pounds ground turkey breast
- 1 piece of sun-dried tomatoes, drained and chopped
- ¼ cup fresh basil leaves, chopped
- 1-oz. low-fat fresh mozzarella, shredded
- ½ teaspoon garlic powder
- ¼ teaspoon salt and ½ teaspoon pepper, to taste

DIRECTIONS

1. Preheat oven to 400°F.
2. Beat the egg in a big mixing bowl.
3. Add the remaining ingredients and mix everything with your hands until evenly combined.
4. Spray a 12-cup muffin tin and divide the turkey mixture among the muffin cups, pressing the mix. Cook in the preheated oven till the turkey is well-cooked for about 25–30 minutes.
5. Chill the meatloaves entirely and store them in a container in the fridge for up to 5 days.

Nutritions: *Calories: 149, Protein: 17g, Carbohydrates: 4.5g, Fats: 6g*

96. CHICKEN LO MEIN

PREPARATION: 15 MIN

COOKING: 15 MIN

SERVES: 1

INGREDIENTS

- 1/2 tablespoon + 1/2 teaspoon sesame oil, divided
- 220g boneless. skinless chicken breasts, sliced
- ¼ teaspoon ground black pepper
- 1/4 tablespoon soy sauce
- 1/4 tablespoon oyster sauce
- 1/4 garlic clove, minced
- 1/2 teaspoon fresh ginger root
- 1/2 spring onions, trimmed and sliced with white and green parts separated
- 25g fresh mushrooms, divided
- 1/4 medium red bell pepper, membranes, and seeds removed
- 1/2 medium zucchinis (400g), cut, sliced

DIRECTIONS

1. In a skillet, heat one-teaspoon sesame oil over medium-high heat. Put the shredded chicken, season with black pepper, and cook until chicken is done (internal temperature about 165°F). Dismiss from wok or skillet and set aside.
2. While the chicken cooks, prepare the sauce by combining the oyster sauce, soy sauce, and two tablespoons sesame oil in a bowl and whisking together. Set aside.
3. With the same skillet used to cook the chicken, heat one teaspoon sesame oil and put the garlic, ginger, and white spring onion pieces; cook until fragrant, about 1 minute. Put the mushrooms and bell peppers and continue to cook until just tender, about 3 minutes. Add zucchini noodles and toss to combine.
4. Pour in the sauce and put the chicken; cook until zucchini is tender, and the mixture should be heated by about 3 to 5 minutes.
5. Garnish with green parts of spring onions.

Nutritions: *Calories: 330, Protein: 48g, Carbohydrates: 9g, Fats: 10g*

97. SHEET PAN CHICKEN FAJITA LETTUCE WRAPS

PREPARATION: 10 MIN

COOKING: 30 MIN

SERVES: 1

INGREDIENTS

- 1/2 b. chicken breast, thinly sliced into strips
- 1/2 bell peppers, thinly sliced into strips
- 1/2 teaspoon olive oil
- 1/2 teaspoon fajita seasoning
- Juice of half a lime
- 1 leaf from a romaine heart
- Optional ¼ cup plain non-fat Greek yogurt

DIRECTIONS

1. Preheat oven to about 400 °F.
2. Merge every ingredient except for lettuce in a big, re-sealable plastic bag. Stir well, make sure to coat chicken and vegetables with oil and seasoning equally.
3. Release contents of the bag equally on a foil-lined baking sheet. Cook for 30 minutes until the chicken is well cooked.
4. Serve on lettuce leaves, topped with Greek yogurt.

Nutritions: *Calories: 352, Protein: 20g, Carbohydrates: 4.1g, Fats: 12g*

98. CAULIFLOWER PIZZA WITH CHICKEN AND TZATZIKI

PREPARATION: 10 MIN | COOKING: 60 MIN | SERVES: 1

INGREDIENTS

- 1 cup rice cauliflower
- 1/2 egg
- 1/2 tablespoon low-fat parmesan cheese
- ¼ teaspoon salt, divided
- 1/4 pound boneless, skinless chicken breast, cut into fine strips
- 2 kalamata olives, pitted and chopped
- ½ teaspoon Italian seasoning
- ¼ teaspoon ground black pepper
- 1/4 cup reduced-fat, shredded mozzarella
- ½ cup peeled, seeded, and grated cucumber
- ½ cup low-fat plain Greek yogurt
- ½ teaspoon crushed garlic

DIRECTIONS

1. Shed the cauliflower "rice" on a baking tin lined with parchment paper and cook at 425 °F for about 30 minutes.
2. Dismiss from the oven and allow to cool.
3. In a paper towel, crush the cauliflower to remove any excess moisture.
4. In a big bowl, combine cauliflower with the parmesan cheese, eggs, and a quarter teaspoon salt. Stir to make a cohesive mix.
5. Put the cauliflower mixture onto the parchment-lined baking tin and press into a 12-inch circle shaped like a pizza.
6. Add the chicken strips, pepper, Italian seasoning, and olives, and toss to combine.
7. Place chicken strips and olives on top of the cauliflower crust and spread with mozzarella cheese. Cook at about 430 °F for 20–25 minutes.
8. While the pizza bakes, make the tzatziki sauce. Combine the grated cucumbers, garlic, yogurt, and a quarter teaspoon of salt.
9. Slice the cauliflower pizza into four wedges and top each wedge with tzatziki.

Nutritions: *Calories: 310, Protein: 50g, Carbohydrates: 11g, Fats: 12g*

99. CHICKEN CHILI

PREPARATION: 10 MIN

COOKING: 30 MIN

SERVES: 1

INGREDIENTS

- 1(¼ pound) boneless chicken breast, cut into bite-size pieces
- 1/4 tablespoon olive oil
- 1/4 cup green spring onion, diced
- 1/3 cup bell pepper, seeded and chopped
- ½ cup jalapenos, seeded and diced
- ½ cloves garlic, minced
- ½ teaspoon salt
- 1/4 teaspoon ground cumin
- 1/4 teaspoon coriander
- 1 cup chicken broth
- 1/2 cup water
- ½(7-oz.) cans green chilies
- 1 tablespoon thick canned coconut milk, chopped green onions, and coriander for garnish

DIRECTIONS

1. Mince the chicken and veggies. Then place a big pot over medium-high heat. Put the peppers, oil, onions, jalapeno, and garlic up.
2. Sauté for 5 minutes, then put the chicken, spices, and salt. Sauté additional 5–8 minutes until chicken is cooked well. Place the green chilies, broth, and coconut milk.
3. Bring to the boil. Cook for 15–20 minutes and shred chicken. Serve topped with green onions and coriander.

Nutritions: *Calories: 226, Protein: 20g, Carbohydrates: 19g, Fats: 8g*

100. EGGPLANT PARMESAN WITH CHOPS

PREPARATION: 5 MIN

COOKING: 40 MIN

SERVES: 1

INGREDIENTS

- Bell peppers any color
- Mushrooms
- Vegetable broth
- Cooking spray
- Pepper
- Salt
- 1/2 packet optavia pancake mix
- 1/3 large eggplant
- Parmesan cheese
- Pork chops

DIRECTIONS

1. Using a non-stick pan, fry the pork chops. You should be using the cooking spray, then spray for 7 minutes each side.
2. You also need to spray the glass cooking pan and lay chops on the bottom.
3. Followed by bell peppers around chops.
4. Put the mushrooms around chops.
5. Next, place vegetable broth over chops filling the pan 1/4 inch from the bottom.
6. Put it in the oven and bake at 350 degrees for 30 minutes.
7. Make sure to peel the eggplant and slice.
8. Mix pancake batter as directed and add 1/8 teaspoon baking powder and two egg whites.
9. Then, mix and dip eggplant in batter fry until golden brown, set aside.
10. Remove chops from oven let cool.
11. Arrange 1/2 cup eggplant and 5-oz. peppers on a plate, scoop 1/4 cup marinara on top of the pork chop.
12. Top with 1/4 cup parmesan cheese.
13. Enjoy! It makes three green servings and one lean serving. Mushroom is an extra 1/2 cup; otherwise, just use it for flavor—put in the microwave for 30 seconds, serve hot.

Nutritions: *Calories: 250, Carbohydrates: 14.5g, Fats: 15.9g, Protein: 25g*

101. SPICY TILAPIA WITH SPINACH

PREPARATION: 10 MIN

COOKING: 30 MIN

SERVES: 1

INGREDIENTS

- 3 cups (1 small bunch) fresh spinach
- 9 oz. raw tilapia (should yield one (7 oz) cooked serving)
- 2 teaspoon olive oil or canola oil
- 1 cup or 2 small (2–2/5") canned tomatoes, make sure to chopped (to lessen the sodium content, you should make use of "no salt" canned tomatoes or fresh tomatoes)
- ¾ teaspoon paprika
- ¼ teaspoon red pepper flakes
- ¼ teaspoon garlic powder
- ½ teaspoon hot sauce

DIRECTIONS

1. Begin by preheating the oven to 350 or 380° F.
2. Then paprika, red pepper flakes, garlic powder, and hot sauce.
3. Brush olive oil all over the fish.
4. Use seasoning mixture to coat the fish. Then place the tilapia flat in a baking pan.
5. Drain juice from canned tomatoes, place tomatoes on top of tilapia.
6. You need to cut the spinach into bite-sized pieces, place around tilapia in the pan.
7. Bake 30 minutes or until tilapia can be easily flaked with a fork and is opaque.

Nutritions: Calories: 350, Protein: 51g, Carbohydrates: 10g, Fats: 10g

102. TERIYAKI HALIBUT

PREPARATION: 5 MIN

COOKING: 10 MIN

SERVES: 1

INGREDIENTS

- 2–¼ cups cabbage, chopped
- 1 cup (1 small) zucchini, chopped
- 1 teaspoon Olive oil
- (7 oz.) raw halibut (should yield one 6-oz cooked serving)
- 2 tablespoon teriyaki sauce
- ½ teaspoon cayenne pepper
- Dash of salt and pepper (optional)

DIRECTIONS

1. Start with sprinkling halibut with cayenne pepper or paprika and baste with teriyaki sauce. Next will be broiling it on tin foil 4" under preheated broiler 7 minutes.
2. Next, we will remove it in the oven and wrap in tin foil until ready to serve (this will continue to cook halibut).
3. Vegetables: Chop up zucchini and cabbage. Sauté olive oil, zucchini, and cabbage in a pan until slightly brown.
4. If desired, season it with salt and pepper to taste. Place on a plate and serve halibut on top of vegetables.

Nutritions: *Calories: 510, Protein: 42.7g, Carbohydrates: 56.7g, Fats: 12.2g*

103. SPICED CROCKPOT ROAST BEEF

PREPARATION: 20 MIN

COOKING: 4-8 H

SERVES: 1

INGREDIENTS

- 1 tablespoon water
- 1/2 tablespoon black pepper
- 1/2 pounds raw, boneless beef chuck clod roast (this should result in six 5-oz cooked servings)
- 1/4 tablespoon soy sauce
- 1 teaspoon balsamic vinegar
- 1/2 teaspoon worcestershire sauce
- 1/2 teaspoon dry mustard
- ½ teaspoon salt or salt substitute
- 1/2 cloves garlic, minced
- 1/2 cups celery, roughly diced
- 3/4 cups green beans, trimmed
- 1/6 cups whole mushrooms, trimmed
- 2 cups scallions, roughly chopped

DIRECTIONS

1. Trim all visible fat from roast. Then rub black pepper and garlic onto roast.
2. Then produce several small shallow slits on top of the roast. Combine remaining spice blend ingredients in a bowl; pour over meat.
3. Then let it cook on low 8–10 hours or high 4–5 hours.
4. Lastly, add vegetables during the last 30–60 minutes of roasting.

Nutritions: *Calories: 180, Protein: 24.7g, Carbohydrates: 14g, Fats: 5g*

104. SPICY GARLIC LIME SHRIMP

PREPARATION: 10 MIN

COOKING: 15 MIN

SERVES: 1

INGREDIENTS

- 1 small 2–½" x 2" chopped green peppers
- ½ tablespoon lime juice
- 1/¾ pound (28 oz.) large, peeled, and deveined raw shrimp, peeled, and deveined; if using frozen, if you choose to use fully cooked shrimp, you need to use 1–1/3 lbs. (about 21 oz.) (both portions should yield three (7 oz) servings)
- 1 cup (2 small 2–2/5") fresh or canned tomatoes, diced (if using canned tomatoes, drain liquid)
- ½ tablespoon olive oil
- 8 oz. packages of hair noodles
- ½ clove garlic, pressed

Seasoning blend:

- ¼ teaspoon salt or salt substitute
- ¼ teaspoon ground black pepper
- ¼ teaspoon cayenne pepper
- ¼ teaspoon dried parsley flakes
- ¼ teaspoon garlic powder
- ¼ teaspoon paprika
- 1/8 teaspoon dried thyme
- 1/8 teaspoon onion powder

DIRECTIONS

1. When you are using frozen shrimp, thaw. Also, devein and peel shrimp.
2. To make the seasoning blend, combine all the spices.
3. Drain liquid from noodles and rinse thoroughly, set aside.
4. Next is preheating a large skillet over medium heat. Once the pan is heated, add olive oil, and stir in pressed garlic cup. Immediately add shrimp, green bell peppers, and lime juice.
5. Make sure to sprinkle the entire seasoning blend over shrimp and peppers.
6. Stir. Sauté shrimp and peppers 3–6 minutes.
7. They were followed by adding the drained noodles. You may continue to cook shrimp, peppers, and noodles. Wait for an additional 2–4 minutes or until shrimp begins to brown and peppers are al dente (tender-crisp).
8. Remove from heat, toss with tomatoes.

Nutritions: *Calories: 529, Protein: 34g, Carbohydrates: 68g, Fats: 13g*

105. ITALIAN SHRIMP AND BROCCOLI

PREPARATION: 5 MIN

COOKING: 15 MIN

SERVES: 1

INGREDIENTS

- 2 cups raw chopped broccoli
- (7 oz.) frozen and cooked shrimp (When cooked, each serving should yield one (7 oz))
- ½ cup (4 medium) cherry tomatoes, chopped
- 2 tablespoon of Lite Northern Italian with Basil & Romano
- ½ teaspoon freshly ground black pepper
- 1 tablespoon parmesan cheese, you may need it to be grated or shredded (optional condiment)
- 1 teaspoon olive oil

DIRECTIONS

1. Thaw frozen shrimp. Just follow the directions on the package (about 5–7 minutes). In a skillet, heat olive oil and add broccoli and chopped cherry tomatoes; sauté until vegetables are al dente (tender-crisp).
2. Remove from heat, cover, and set aside. Spoon salad dressing into a skillet; add shrimp and black pepper. Sauté until shrimp are cooked (or opaque in color).
3. Combine shrimp and vegetables; cook an additional 2–3 minutes to reheat vegetables, if necessary. Place shrimp and vegetables on a plate, add parmesan cheese (optional condiment), and stir.

Nutritions: *Calories: 529, Protein: 34g, Carbohydrates: 68g, Fats: 13g*

106. PAN-"FRIED" CATFISH

PREPARATION: 5 MIN

COOKING: 10 MIN

SERVES: 1

INGREDIENTS

- 1–½ cups (½ large) summer squash, sliced
- 8 oz. wild catfish, raw, you may also opt for 6 oz. farmed catfish, raw (This should result in one 7-oz cooked wild catfish providing or one 5-oz cooked farmed catfish serving)
- Non-stick cooking spray
- 1–½ cups (1 small-medium) zucchini, sliced
- 1/2 teaspoon olive oil
- 1/2 tablespoon low-fat mayonnaise, like Miracle Whip® or Kraft® light mayonnaise
- 1/3 teaspoon coriander leaves, chopped
- 1/2 teaspoon lime juice
- 1/16 teaspoon chili powder or ground chipotle chile pepper

DIRECTIONS

1. Start with the tartar sauce by mixing mayonnaise, coriander, lime juice, and chili powder/chipotle pepper in a bowl.
2. Make sure to mix well; set aside for later use. Clean and chop zucchini and squash. Lightly brush catfish with olive oil.
3. Now, preheat a small non-stick skillet on medium-high heat. Later spray the skillet with non-stick cooking spray can for 5–10 seconds.
4. Then, sauté the chopped vegetables until al dente (tender-crisp). Do not forget to remove vegetables from heat and cover-up to keep warm while cooking catfish. Place catfish (brushed with olive oil) in the pan, let it cook each side for 1 minute or until seared.
5. Next, lessen the heat to medium. Let it cook 2–3 minutes on each side or until catfish flakes easily, use a fork. Lastly, serve cooked catfish with sautéed vegetables.

Nutritions: *Calories: 151, Protein: 26g, Carbohydrates: 0g, Fats: 4.5g*

107. ZESTY GRILLED VEGETABLES AND MAHI-MAHI

PREPARATION: 5 MIN

COOKING: 15 MIN

SERVES: 1

INGREDIENTS

- 1 pound (16 oz.) raw mahi-mahi (should yield two (7 oz) cooked servings)
- 1 cup (1 small) zucchini with peel, sliced
- 1 cup (1 medium-large 3" x 2–¾") red bell pepper, sliced
- 1 cup (1 medium-large 3" x 2–¾") yellow bell pepper, sliced
- ¼ cup Newman's Own® Family Recipe Italian Dressing
- 1 serving of green

DIRECTIONS

1. Preheat grill to medium heat. Place vegetables in a grill basket.
2. Grill 10 minutes or until al dente (tender-crisp), turning occasionally.
3. Then place fish on the grill and cook for 4–5 minutes on each side. You may also wait until fish flakes easily with a fork.
4. Next, place vegetables in a medium bowl. Also, add the dressing. You need to toss it for coating.
5. Divide the vegetables onto two plates and place one serving of mahi-mahi on each plate.

Nutritions: *Calories: 340, Protein: 50g, Carbohydrates: 14g, Fats: 10g*

108. REFRESHING TILAPIA

PREPARATION: 5 MIN

COOKING: 15 MIN

SERVES: 1

INGREDIENTS

- (8 oz.) wild and raw catfish or (6 oz.) farmed catfish, natural (should yield one (7 oz) cooked wild catfish serving or one (5 oz) cooked farmed catfish serving)
- 1–½ cups (½ large) sliced summer squash
- 1–½ cups (1 small-medium) sliced zucchini
- 1 teaspoon olive oil
- Non-stick cooking spray
- 1 tablespoon low-fat mayonnaise
- 1/8 teaspoon chili powder
- 1–½ teaspoon chopped coriander leaves
- 1 teaspoon lime juice

DIRECTIONS

1. Prepare the tartar sauce by combining mayonnaise, coriander, lime juice, and chili powder/chipotle pepper in a small bowl. Mix well; set aside for later use.
2. Next will be cleaning and chopping zucchini and squash. Then make sure to brush catfish with olive oil lightly.
3. The next thing to do is to preheat a small non-stick skillet over medium-high heat. Then spray the skillet with non-stick cooking spray for 5–10 seconds.
4. The next step is to sauté chopped vegetables until al dente (tender-crisp). Do not forget to eliminate vegetables from heat and cover to keep warm while cooking catfish.
5. Place catfish (brushed with olive oil) in the pan, let it cook for 1 minute on each side.
6. Cook 2–3 minutes on each side, or you may wait until the catfish flakes easily with a fork. Serve cooked catfish with sautéed vegetables.

Nutritions: *Calories: 350, Protein: 51g, Carbohydrates: 10g, Fats: 10g*

109. SUN-DRIED TOMATO SHRIMP

PREPARATION: 5 MIN | COOKING: 15 MIN | SERVES: 1

INGREDIENTS

- 8 oz. raw shrimp, peeled, and deveined, you may also opt for (7 oz.) fully cooked frozen shrimp, thawed (either starting portion should yield one (7 oz) cooked serving)
- 1 cup romaine lettuce, chopped or shredded
- ½ cup (1 medium 2–3/5") tomato, diced
- ½ cup cucumber, sliced
- 4 tablespoon Newman's ® Lighten Up Sun-Dried Tomato Dressing, divided

DIRECTIONS

1. Marinate shrimp in 3 tablespoon Newman's ® Lighten Up Sun-Dried Tomato Dressing for 1–2 hours.
2. Prepare the salad by washing vegetables and cutting them as indicated above; set aside. After shrimp has sufficiently marinated, pour entire contents (shrimp and marinade) into a skillet and cook over medium heat until shrimp are cooked through (or turn opaque in color) 3–5 minutes.
3. Then drizzle 1 tablespoon Newman's ® Lighten Up Sun-Dried Tomato Dressing over.

Nutritions: *Calories: 529, Protein: 34g, Carbohydrates: 68g, Fats: 13g*

110. FALL CHICKEN NOODLE STIR FRY

PREPARATION: 5 MIN

COOKING: 10 MIN

SERVES: 1

INGREDIENTS

- 2 oz. chicken breast
- 1/4 cup butternut squash cubes
- 1 egg, whole,
- 1 oz. of brown rice pad thai noodles
- 1/2 tablespoon of fish sauce
- 1/4 teaspoon sesame oil, untoasted
- 1/4 tablespoon of Teriyaki sauce
- 1/4 tablespoon of sriracha
- 1/2 teaspoon of garlic
- 1 serving of fresh bean sprouts
- 1 lean
- 2 green
- 1 condiment

DIRECTIONS

1. First, cook the noodles as indicated by the package.
2. In the microwave, eat up the pre-cooked butternut squash.
3. The next step is cooking for 3–5 minutes, or you may opt to wait when the squash softens.
4. Meanwhile, in a non-stick skillet, heat the oil over medium heat. Then add the garlic, chicken, and butternut squash. You may cut up the chicken in the skillet and heat until golden.
5. Scramble the eggs to the skillet. Wait for the noodles to become 75%–80% cooked through. You may now add the noodles to the skillet. It may be followed by adding the fish sauce, teriyaki sauce, and sriracha. Stir often.
6. Proceed by adding the bean sprouts. Cook for an additional minute to two until bean sprouts are heated. Serve on a bowl.
7. If desired, top with red pepper flakes and coriander.

Nutritions: *Protein: 51g, Calories: 350, Carbohydrates: 10g, Fats: 10g*

111. HEALTHY SALMON CHOWDER

PREPARATION: 10 MIN

COOKING: 10 MIN

SERVES: 1

INGREDIENTS

- 1/4 tablespoon olive oil
- 1/4 small onion, diced
- 1/4 cup chopped coriander leaves or stems
- ½ chipotle peppers in adobo, diced
- 1/2 medium head of cauliflower, chopped
- 1/2 cups chicken broth (low sodium)
- 1 cup baby spinach
- 1/4 cup frozen corn
- 4 oz. salmon
- 1 oz. low-fat Greek yogurt
- Finishing salt
- Chili flakes

DIRECTIONS

1. Heat oil, chopped onion, coriander stems, and sauté until brown, 3 to 4 minutes.
2. Add chipotle peppers and cauliflower. Cook for 1 to 2 minutes.
3. You may now add the chicken broth and wait for it to simmer.
4. Wait for it to cook for 5 minutes, or until cauliflower is tender.
5. Over medium-high heat adds spinach and corn. Let cook for 1 to 2 minutes.
6. Crumble salmon to bite-size chunk then add to the pot.
7. Reduce heat to a gentle simmer.
8. Do not forget to remove from heat and stir in Greek yogurt.
9. Finally, serve warm with finishing salt and chili flakes if desired.

Nutritions: *Calories: 350, Protein: 51g, Carbohydrates: 10g, Fats: 10g*

112. FLAT IRON STEAK FAJITA BOWLS

PREPARATION: 5 MIN

COOKING: 5 MIN

SERVES: 1

INGREDIENTS

- 4 oz. flat iron steak
- Fresh coriander
- 1/4 cup white corn
- 1/2 yellow onion
- 1/2 cup bell peppers
- 1/2 cup brown rice
- Green leaf lettuce
- Jalapenos (optional)
- Red pepper flakes
- Avocado (optional)

DIRECTIONS

1. Cut the onion and combine bell peppers.
2. Next, cut the flat iron steak into strips.
3. Heat a skillet and then spray with non-stick spray.
4. Grill the steak and vegetables until cooked.
5. Heat two cups of brown rice in a microwave. (For best results, place a wet paper towel on top of the bowl of rice before heating).
6. Drain the can of corn and rinse.
7. On a plate, portion out the base layer of rice, steak, fajita veggies.
8. If desired, top with lettuce, corn, jalapenos, and red pepper flakes.

Nutritions: *Calories: 352, Protein: 20g, Carbohydrates: 4.1g, Fats: 12g*

113. REAL SIMPLE AND CLEAN MEATBALLS

PREPARATION: 5 MIN

COOKING: 25 MIN

SERVES: 1

INGREDIENTS

- 1/2 pounds of lean grass-fed ground beef
- 1/2 medium onion
- 1 clove garlic
- 1 egg
- 1/4 cup quinoa flour
- Salt and pepper to taste

DIRECTIONS

1. Preheat your oven to 350°F.
2. Then, cut the onion into small pieces, add the minced garlic
3. Next will be adding the meat, onion, garlic, egg, quinoa flour, salt, and pepper in a large mixing bowl and mix until well combined.
4. Next, using your hands, grab a small amount of the meat mixture and work into a ball, about 1 inch in diameter.
5. Put the meatball on a baking sheet that has been sprayed with nonstick spray. Then repeat this process with the remaining meat mixture. It should yield about 25 meatballs.
6. Lastly, put the meatballs in the oven for 25 minutes. Serve with your favorite sauce and veggies!

Nutritions: *Calories: 350, Protein: 51g, Carbohydrates: 10g, Fats: 10g*

114. HIGH PROTEIN LOW CARB SHRIMP CEVICHE

PREPARATION: 5 MIN

COOKING: 1 MIN

SERVES: 1

INGREDIENTS

- 1 (5-oz.) package shrimp
- 1/2 red bell pepper
- 1/2 small cucumber
- 1 to 2 radishes
- 1/2 large tomato
- 1/4 jalapeno
- 1/8 cup fresh coriander, diced (Stems and Leaves)
- 1/4 tablespoon olive oil
- ½ lime, juice, and zest
- 1/4 teaspoon salt

DIRECTIONS

1. Start to dice all veggies into bite-size. Finely chop coriander stems and leaves, leaving some leaves for garnish.
2. Mix the oil with lime juice, lime zest, salt, and coriander in a bowl. Make sure to add a dash of honey or sugar if needed for taste.
3. Make sure to drain shrimp and mix it in a bowl with veggies.
4. Last, toss shrimp and veggies in the coriander dressing and serve.

Nutritions: *Calories: 529, Protein: 34g, Carbohydrates: 68g, Fats: 13g*

115. STEAK AND AVOCADO LETTUCE WRAPS

PREPARATION: 15 MIN

COOKING: 20 MIN

SERVES: 4-8 WRAPS

INGREDIENTS

- 1 pound steak, diced
- 1 large head butter, bibb, or boston lettuce, washed, pat dried and leaves separated
- 2 mediums avocado
- 1/2 cup favorite salsa, store-bought
- 1/2 teaspoon Kosher Salt
- 1/2 teaspoon black pepper
- 1 tablespoon coriander seed
- 1/2 teaspoon garlic powder
- 1 tablespoon coconut oil
- Favorite toppings of choice

DIRECTIONS

1. Wash, dry, and separate the leaves of the chosen green. We recommend using butter lettuce, but any large leaf lettuce that you enjoy will work. Set aside.
2. Dice your choice of protein. In a pan, heat coconut oil over medium-low heat and add the spices to the oil.
3. Slightly toast the spices until aromatic. Increase the heat to medium-high, and make sure not to burn the spices, add the diced protein. Sauté for 3–5 minutes, until the protein is warm.
4. In a small bowl, mash the flesh of two avocados with a fork until just creamy. Add salt and lime juice to taste if desired. Spread avocado into each piece of lettuce.
5. Equally, distribute protein onto the lettuce wraps and top with favorite salsa to taste. Fold like a taco and enjoy!
6. Use any favorite toppings like chopped tomatoes, diced onions, and coriander!

Nutritions: *Calories: 250, Carbohydrates: 14.5g, Fats: 15.9g, Protein: 25g*

116. BEST INSTANT POT VEGGIE CHILI

PREPARATION: 15 MIN

COOKING: 30 MIN

SERVES: 1

INGREDIENTS

- 1/8 large onion chopped
- 1/8 red bell pepper diced
- 1/8 green bell pepper diced
- 3/8 cloves garlic minced
- 1 oz. Seitan optional
- 1/2 cups Cauliflower crumb optional
- 1 oz. Mushrooms optional
- 1/4 cups water
- 1/8 teaspoon garlic powder
- 1/8 teaspoon black pepper
- 1/4 teaspoon paprika
- 1/4 teaspoon oregano
- 1/4 teaspoon chipotle chili powder optional
- 1/2 teaspoon ground cumin
- 1/8 cup chili powder
- 1/3 oz. can pinto beans low sodium
- 1/2 oz. can kidney beans low sodium
- 1/2 oz. can tomato sauce low sodium
- 1/3 oz. can dice tomatoes (fire-roasted)
- 1 (2 oz.) can tomato paste
- 1/4 tablespoon masa tamale flour

DIRECTIONS

1. Chop all vegetables and add to IP.
2. Lightly sauté vegetables in a small amount of water, veg broth, or bean juice (aquafaba) until softened.
3. If using—add seitan, cauliflower crumb, or mushrooms for a meat substitute. Note all of these are optional, and you could just add another can of beans.
4. Add water and all spices, except Masa, and stir well 5. Mix in beans and go well.
5. Followed by adding tomato sauce and diced tomatoes to TOP of stew and DO NOT STIR.
6. Next, add the lid to IP and set it to MANUAL mode for 10 minutes.
7. Allow to naturally vent when completed for 10 minutes before CAREFULLY releasing any additional pressure.
8. Stir in tomato paste, and any last-minute garnishes, and Masa flour.
9. Let rest for 10 minutes to thicken, make sure to stir occasionally.

Nutritions: *Calories: 350, Protein: 51g, Carbohydrates: 10g, Fats: 10g*

117. CHANA MASALA

PREPARATION: 20 MIN

COOKING: 30 MIN

SERVES: 1

INGREDIENTS

- 1/4 onion, chopped
- 1/4 garlic clove, sliced
- 1/2 tablespoon chopped peeled ginger
- 1/2 tablespoon vegetable oil
- 1/4 cardamom pods
- 1/4 teaspoon curry powder
- 1 (7 oz.) can be peeled whole tomatoes with their juices, crushed
- 1 (3 oz.) can chickpeas, rinsed
- Kosher salt and freshly ground black pepper
- Cooked basmati rice (for serving)
- Chopped fresh coriander (for serving)

DIRECTIONS

1. Cook onion, garlic, and ginger with cardamom and curry powder until onion is soft, 8–10 minutes.
2. Then add tomatoes with their juices and chickpeas and simmer until soft, 25–30-minute, season with salt and pepper.
3. Serve with rice and coriander.

Nutritions: *Calories: 350, Protein: 51g, Carbohydrates: 10g, Fats: 10g*

118. TURKEY STUFFED BELL PEPPERS

PREPARATION: 10 MIN

COOKING: 25 MIN

SERVES: 1

INGREDIENTS

- 1 Whole bell peppers (We used Red & Green)
- 1 (4 oz.) turkey burger
- 1/8 red onion (diced)
- 1/2 medium tomato (chopped)
- 1/4 cup panko breadcrumbs
- 1/4 cup low-fat shredded cheddar cheese
- 1/2 teaspoon Italian seasoning
- 1/2 teaspoon ground cumin
- 1/2 clove garlic
- Salt and pepper

DIRECTIONS

1. Preheat oven to 325 degrees. Then, cut the bell peppers in half, remove seeds, and clean.
2. In a large bowl, crumble the turkey burgers and mix with the onions, breadcrumbs, tomato, garlic, and the seasoning. Next, you need to add half of the cheese to the bowl (save another half for the top). Add a dash of salt and pepper. Mix well together.
3. Spray a baking sheet with non-stick cooking spray.
4. Then add the bell pepper halves. Fill each bell peppers with the stuffing. Heat for 15–20 minutes.
5. Remove the bell peppers from heat and add the rest of the cheese to the top of the peppers. Place back in the oven for 3–5 minutes or until cheese is melted.

Nutritions: *Calories: 350, Protein: 51g, Carbohydrates: 10g, Fats: 10g*

119. LEAN CROCKPOT PULLED PORK

PREPARATION: 15 MIN　COOKING: 480 MIN　SERVES: 1

INGREDIENTS

- 1 Boneless pork chops
- 1/2 (15 oz.) cans tomato sauce, no sugar added
- 1/3 tablespoon onion powder
- 1/2 tablespoon garlic powder
- 1/4 tablespoon cumin
- 1/2 teaspoon cinnamon
- 1/4 teaspoon chili powder
- 1/8 teaspoon cayenne pepper

DIRECTIONS

1. Trim extra fat from pork and add to crockpot.
2. Make sure to add the tomato sauce and seasonings to a bowl and mix.
3. Pour the sauce over the pork chops.
4. Cook for 8 to 12 hours on low heat or until meat is thoroughly tender and starts to fall apart.
5. Lastly, pull the pork apart with a fork and enjoy!

Nutritions: *Calories: 250, Carbohydrates: 14.5g, Fats: 15.9g, Protein: 25g*

120. EASY CREAMY CAJUN SHRIMP PASTA

PREPARATION: 5 MIN

COOKING: 15 MIN

SERVES: 1

INGREDIENTS

- 2 oz. linguine pasta
- 1/4 teaspoon olive oil
- 1/4 pound raw shrimp
- 1/4 tablespoon cajun
- 1 oz. sausage
- 1/8 red peppers
- 1/8 green peppers
- 1/8 onions
- 1/2 tomatoes
- 1/2 tablespoon butter
- 1/2 whip cream
- 1/2 almond milk
- 1 oz. cream cheese
- 1/2 shredded parmesan reggiano

DIRECTIONS

1. Cook the pasta as per package instructions.
2. Place the shrimp in a bowl along with 1/2 tablespoon of cajun or creole seasoning. Mix to ensure the shrimp is fully coated.
3. Heat a skillet or pan on medium-high heat. I use a cast-iron skillet. Next, add 1 teaspoon of olive oil to the pan.
4. While it is hot, add the shrimp to the pan. Then cook each side for 2–3 minutes until it turns bright pink. Remove the shrimp and set aside.
5. The next step will be adding a teaspoon of olive oil to the pan along with the chopped sausage, onions, green peppers, and red peppers.
6. Sauté for 3–4 minutes until the vegetables are soft and the onions are translucent and fragrant. Make sure to remove the vegetables from the pan and set aside.
7. You also need to reduce the heat on the pan to medium. Do not forget to add the butter to the pan and

allow it to melt.

8. The next step will be adding the heavy cream, almond milk, cream cheese, the remaining 1/2 tablespoon of cajun or creole seasoning, and parmesan Reggiano cheese.
9. Just continue stirring the sauce until all the cheese has fully melted. The cream cheeses may take some time to melt. Add in the fire-roasted tomatoes and stir. Allow the mixture to cook for 2 minutes.
10. Next, you need to add the shrimp, sausage, vegetables, and pasta to the pan and stir. Allow the pasta to cook for 4–5 minutes until combined. Serve.

Nutritions: Calories: 384, Protein: 7g, Carbohydrates: 22g, Fats: 28 g

CHAPTER 11: DESSERTS

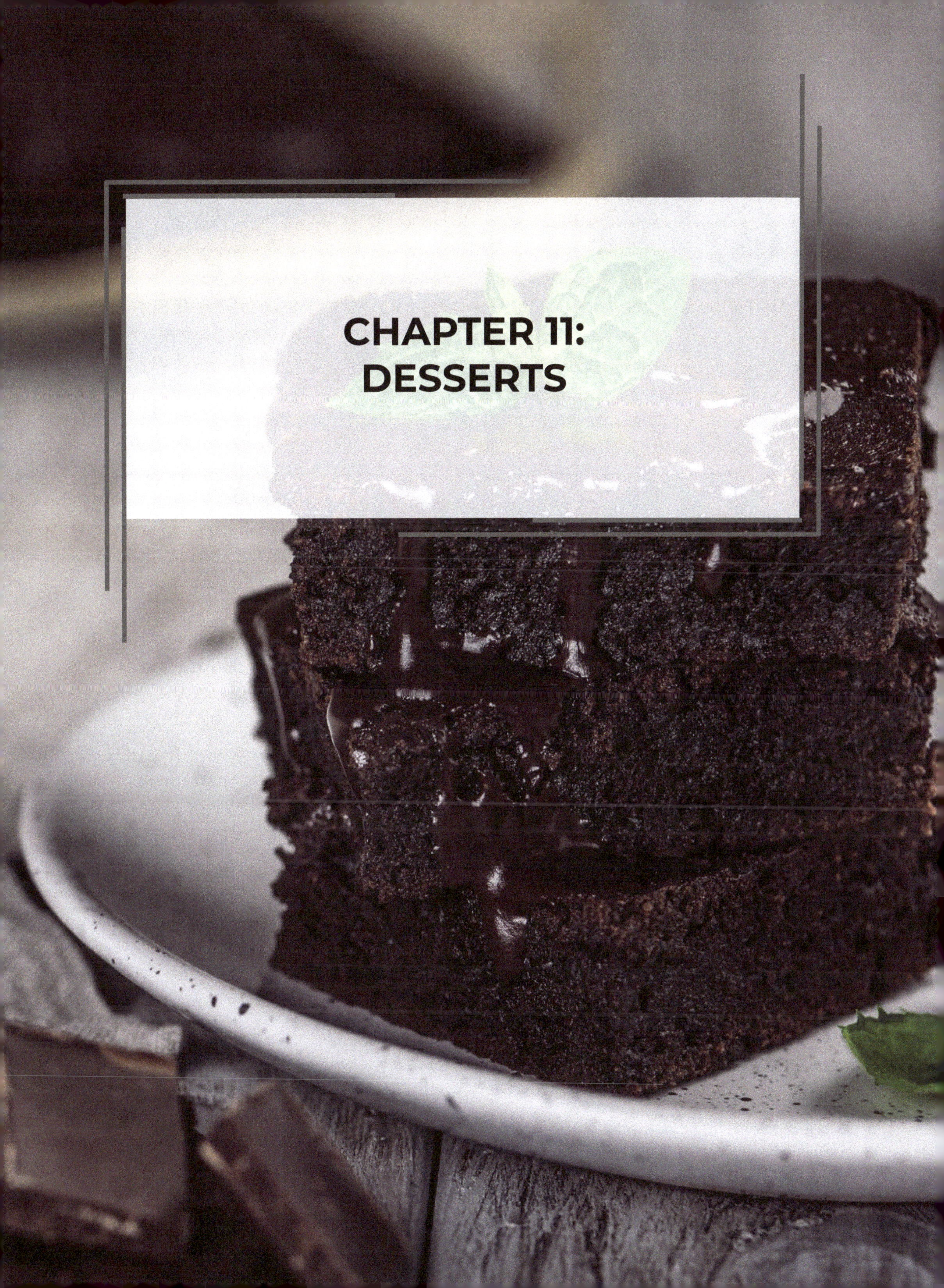

121. TRIPLE CHOCOLATE CHIP DEEP DISH COOKIES

PREPARATION: 10 MIN

COOKING: 30 MIN

SERVES: 1

INGREDIENTS

- 3/4 cup canned pumpkin
- 3/4 cup chocolate peanut butter
- 1/2 cup powdered chocolate protein
- 1/4 cup honey
- 1 beaten egg
- 1 teaspoon pure vanilla
- 1/2 teaspoon baking soda
- 1/2 cup sugar-free chocolate chips
- Vanilla ice cream or serving

DIRECTIONS

1. Add all the ingredients except ice cream and chocolate chips in a bowl
2. Use a mixer (electric) beat until mixed evenly.
3. Heat your oven to 350 degrees Fahrenheit.
4. Gradually add the chocolate chips and gently fold to incorporate.
5. Pour batter into a skillet (medium).
6. Place skillet into a preheated oven to bake for approximately 20 minutes until golden brown.
7. Remove from heat and set aside for roughly 7–10 minutes.
8. Serve using the vanilla ice cream.

Nutritions: *Calories: 502, Protein: 6g, Carbohydrates: 65g, Fats: 24g*

122. PROTEIN BROWNIES

PREPARATION: 10 MIN COOKING: 30-35 MIN SERVES: 1

INGREDIENTS

- 1/2 cup almond milk
- 1/2 cup, chocolate flavored egg whites
- 1/2 cup, unsweetened apple sauce
- 1/2 cup+1 tablespoon Greek yogurt
- 1 cup, oat flour
- 2–3 scoops, powdered chocolate protein
- 3 tablespoon., powdered unsweetened cocoa
- 1 teaspoon, baker style baking powder
- 1/2 teaspoon salt

Ingredients for the frosting:

- 1/2 cup, nonfat Greek yogurt
- 1/4 cup cherries
- Sweetener (optional)

DIRECTIONS

1. The first step is to heat an oven to 350 degrees Fahrenheit then lightly spray a baking dish using cooking spray.
2. Add the egg whites and whisk well until beaten lightly.
3. Add the protein powder, oat flour, sweetener, powdered cocoa, and the baking powder separately.
4. Stir well until mixed evenly, then pour milk mixture (almond) into the flour mixture.
5. Stir well until thoroughly mixed and set batter aside for approximately 5 minutes.
6. Pour batter into the dish and place into the oven to bake for approximately 25 minutes until thoroughly cooked.
7. Remove brownie from heat then set aside to cool.
8. Add all the frosting ingredients in a food processor then process on the highest setting until it becomes smooth.
9. Spread frosting over the top of brownies. Serve.

Nutritions: *Calories: 466, Protein: 6g, Carbohydrates: 50g, Fats: 29g*

123. PROTEIN PUMPKIN SPICED DONUTS

PREPARATION: 10 MIN | COOKING: 15 MIN | SERVES: 1

INGREDIENTS

- 1 cup oat flour
- 3/4 cup xylitol
- 1 scoop, powdered vanilla protein
- 1 tablespoon, ground flaxseed
- 1 tablespoon, ground cinnamon
- 2 teaspoon baking powder
- 1 teaspoon sea salt
- 3 beaten eggs
- 1/2 cup canned pumpkin
- 1 tablespoon melted coconut oil
- 2 teaspoon pure vanilla
- 1 teaspoon apple cider vinegar

Ingredients for the frosting:

- 1/2 cup whipped cream cheese
- 1/2 teaspoon liquid stevia

DIRECTIONS

1. Place the xylitol, oat flour, ground flaxseed, powdered protein, baking powder, ground cinnamon, and a dash of sea salt in a large bowl. Preheat your oven to 350°F.
2. Add the egg (beaten) into another bowl (large) along with the pumpkin (canned), pure vanilla, and vinegar and coconut oil (melted).
3. Whisk until mixed (evenly), then pour the mixture into the flour. Stir until thoroughly mixed.
4. Use cooking spray grease a large donut pan.
5. Pour batter into the donut pan (greased).
6. Place batter into the oven and bake for approximately 10 minutes until thoroughly baked.
7. Remove from heat and set donuts onto a wire rack to cool.
8. Add in the cream cheese (whipped) and liquid stevia in a small bowl, whisk until it becomes smooth.
9. Frost donuts using the frosting and serve with a sprinkle of cinnamon (ground) over the top.

Nutritions: *Calories: 452, Protein: 4.9g, Carbohydrates: 51g, Fats: 25g*

124. HIGH PROTEIN CHIPOTLE CHEDDAR QUESADILLA

PREPARATION: 15 MIN

COOKING: 45 MIN

SERVES: 1

INGREDIENTS

- 1 low carb tortillas
- 1/2 cups low sodium cottage cheese
- 1/2 cups low fat, shredded cheddar cheese
- 1/4 red thinly sliced bell pepper
- 1/4 thinly sliced onion
- 1/4 cup thinly sliced portobello mushrooms
- 1 tablespoon chipotle seasoning
- Mild salsa (for dipping)

DIRECTIONS

1. Add the bell pepper (sliced, red), onion (sliced), and mushrooms (sliced) into a large grill pan over medium heat.
2. Cook for approximately 10 minutes until soft. Remove then transfer into a bowl (medium). Set aside.
3. Add the chipotle seasoning and cottage cheese in a small bowl. Stir well to incorporate.
4. Place tortillas onto the grill pan and pour vegetable mixture over tortillas.
5. Sprinkle cottage cheese mixture over the top then top off using the cheddar cheese (shredded).
6. Place an additional tortilla over the top of the filling.
7. Cook for roughly 2 minutes, then flip and continue cooking for the next minute.
8. Repeat process with remaining tortillas and filling. 9. Serve immediately with the salsa (mild).

Nutritions: *Calories: 293, Protein: 15g, Carbohydrates: 24g, Fats: 15g*

125. SWEET POTATO CASSEROLE

PREPARATION: 5 MIN

COOKING: 15 MIN

SERVES: 1

INGREDIENTS

- 1/2 pounds sweet, peeled, chopped)Potatoes
- 1/3 cup nonfat Greek yogurt
- 1/2 tablespoon ground cinnamon
- 1/8 teaspoon ground nutmeg
- 1/4 teaspoon sea salt
- 1 tablespoon egg whites
- 1/4 tablespoon melted utter
- 1/2 cup chopped pecans
- 1/2 cup miniature marshmallows
- Sugar (dash, light brown, for sprinkling)

DIRECTIONS

1. Heat your oven to 375 degrees Fahrenheit.
2. Place the potatoes (sweet) into a saucepan (large) over medium-high heat.
3. Cover potatoes using water, then bring to a boil, boil for approximately 30 minutes until soft.
4. Drain potatoes, then place potatoes back into the saucepan.
5. Add the Greek yogurt, cinnamon (ground), nutmeg (ground), and sea salt (dash) into the potatoes.
6. Stir well until coated (evenly).
7. Add in the butter (melted) and egg whites then bring to a stir once more.
8. Transfer potato mixture into a casserole dish (large).
9. Place into the oven then bakes for approximately 30 minutes. Remove from heat then top with the pecans (chopped) and miniature marshmallows.
10. Place back into the oven to bake for an additional 10 minutes until marshmallows are browned.

Nutritions: *Calories: 86, Protein: 1.6g, Carbohydrates: 20g, Fats: 0.1g*

126. BARBECUE PULLED PORK SANDWICHES

PREPARATION: 10 MIN

COOKING: 6 H

SERVES: 1

INGREDIENTS

- ¼ pound pork tenderloin
- 1/4 cup barbecue sauce
- 1 hamburger rolls
- 1/2 cup shredded coleslaw
- 1/2 cup Greek yogurt
- 1 ½ tablespoon dijon mustard
- Salt and black pepper (dash)

DIRECTIONS

1. Add in the pork tenderloin into a slow cooker then pour barbecue sauce over the top.
2. Cover using the lid and cook for 6 hours on medium setting until soft.
3. Remove pork tenderloin and finely shred using two forks.
4. Add in the yogurt, coleslaw, and Dijon mustard into a small-sized bowl and season using a dash of salt and black pepper. Stir until thoroughly mixed.
5. Divide pork among hamburger buns then tops off using the coleslaw.
6. Serve immediately.

Nutritions: *Calories: 155, Protein: 34g, Carbohydrates: 28g, Fats: 10g*

127. SWEET CINNAMON ROLLS

PREPARATION: 10 MIN

COOKING: 20 MIN

SERVES: 1

INGREDIENTS

Dough:

- ¼ cup Oat flour extra for rolling
- 1 tablespoon coconut sugar
- 1 teaspoon baking powder
- ½ teaspoon xanthium gum
- 1/2 tablespoon cold coconut oil
- 1 to 2 tablespoon whole milk

Filling:

- 1 tablespoon melted coconut oil
- ½ tablespoon ground cinnamon
- 2 tablespoon coconut sugar

Ingredients for the frosting:

- ¼ cup Greek yogurt
- 1 to 2 tablespoon whole milk
- 1 tablespoon vanilla protein
- Pecans

DIRECTIONS

1. Preheat the oven to 400°F.
2. In a bowl (large), put in all the ingredients for the dough. Stir thoroughly to mix until your dough becomes soft. Before putting it into the fridge, cover the dough and allow chill for about 20 minutes.
3. Put the dough onto a flat surface that has been dusted with flour. Roll the dough into a square (large).
4. Spread half of the coconut oil over the top part of the dough. Use coconut sugar and ground cinnamon to sprinkle over the top.
5. Using jelly-roll style, roll the dough. Slice the dough into rolls. Place onto a baking sheet (large) with the side that was cut facing down.
6. Spread the coconut oil over the top of the rolls.
7. Place cinnamon rolls into the oven to bake for approximately 20 minutes. 8. For 10 minutes, let it cool, then serve.

Nutritions: Calories: 436, Protein: 4.7g, Carbohydrates: 50g, Fats: 24g

128. PUFFED BROWN RICE

PREPARATION: 5 MIN

COOKING: 15 MIN

SERVES: 1

INGREDIENTS

- 1/4 cup dry and brown rice
- 1–2 cups MCT oil

DIRECTIONS

1. Use paper towels to line a medium bowl.
2. In a saucepan, pour 5–8 cups of MCT oil and heat over medium-high heat.
3. Ensure that saucepan is fully covered with oil.
4. Once the oil is hot enough, place the rice grains (dry) using a sieve until the pot is fully covered with rice.
5. Gently shake to ensure everything puffs up. Be careful not to burn the rice.
6. Remove sieve with the rice (puffed) then transfer puffed grains into the bowl.
7. Set aside to let cool, then discard the leftover oil. 8. Once cooled. Enjoy.

Nutritions: *Calories: 402, Protein: 6g, Carbohydrates: 90g, Fats: 0.5g*

129. HOMEMADE CHOCOLATES WITH COCONUT AND RAISINS

PREPARATION: 10 MIN | COOKING: CHILLING TIME | SERVES: 1

INGREDIENTS

- 1/2 cup cacao butter, melted
- 1/3 cup peanut butter
- 1/4 cup agave syrup
- A pinch of grated nutmeg
- A bit of coarse salt
- 1/2 teaspoon vanilla extract
- 1 cup dried coconut, shredded
- 6 oz. dark chocolate, chopped
- 3 oz. raisins

DIRECTIONS

1. Carefully combine all the ingredients, not including for the chocolate, in a mixing bowl.
2. Spoon the mixture into molds. Leave to set hard in a cool place.
3. Melt the dark chocolate in your microwave. Pour in the melted chocolate until the fillings are covered. Leave to set hard in a cool place.
4. Enjoy!

Nutritions: Calories: 130, Fat: 9.1g, Carbs: 12.1g, Protein: 1.3g

130. EASY MOCHA FUDGE

PREPARATION: 10 MIN

COOKING: 60 MIN

SERVES: 1

INGREDIENTS

- 1 cup cookies, crushed
- 1/2 cup almond butter
- 1/4 cup agave nectar
- 6 oz. dark chocolate, broken into chunks
- 1 teaspoon instant coffee
- A pinch grated nutmeg
- A pinch salt

DIRECTIONS

1. Line a large baking layer with parchment paper.
2. Melt the chocolate in your microwave and add in the remaining ingredients; stir to combine well.
3. Scrape the batter into a parchment-lined baking sheet. Put it in your freezer for a minimum of 1 hour to set.
4. Cut into squares and serve. Bon appétit!

Nutritions: *Calories: 105, Fat: 5.6g, Carbs: 12.9g, Protein: 1.1g*

131. ALMOND AND CHOCOLATE CHIP BARS

PREPARATION: 10 MIN

COOKING: 30 MIN

SERVES: 1

INGREDIENTS

- 1/2 cup almond butter
- 1/4 cup coconut oil, melted
- 1/4 cup agave syrup
- 1 teaspoon vanilla extract
- 1/4 teaspoon sea salt
- 1/4 teaspoon grated nutmeg
- 1/2 teaspoon ground cinnamon
- 2 cups almond flour
- 1/4 cup flaxseed meal
- 1 cup vegan chocolate, cut into chunks
- 1 1/3 cups almonds, ground
- 2 tablespoons cacao powder
- 1/4 cup agave syrup

DIRECTIONS

1. In a mixing bowl, thoroughly combine the almond butter, coconut oil, 1/4 cup of agave syrup, vanilla, salt, nutmeg, and cinnamon.
2. Gradually stir in the almond flour and flaxseed meal and stir to combine. Add in the chocolate chunks and start again.
3. In a small blending bowl, combine the almonds, cacao powder, and agave syrup. Now, spread the ganache onto the cake. Freeze for about 30 minutes, cut into bars, and serve well chilled. Enjoy!

Nutritions: *Calories: 295, Fat: 17g, Carbs: 35.2g, Protein: 1.7g*

132. ALMOND BUTTER COOKIES

PREPARATION: 10 MIN

COOKING: 30 MIN

SERVES: 1

INGREDIENTS

- 3/4 cup all-purpose flour
- 1/2 teaspoon baking soda
- 1/4 teaspoon kosher salt
- 1 flax egg
- 1/4 cup coconut grease, at room temperature
- 2 tablespoons almond milk
- 1/2 cup brown sugar
- 1/2 cup almond butter
- 1/2 teaspoon ground cinnamon
- 1/2 teaspoon vanilla

DIRECTIONS

1. In a blending bowl, blend the flour, baking soda, and salt.
2. In another bowl, combine the flax egg, coconut oil, almond milk, sugar, almond butter, cinnamon, and vanilla. Whisk the wet mixture into the dry materials and stir until well combined.
3. Place the batter in your refrigerator for just about 30 minutes. Form the batter into small cookies and assemble them on a parchment-lined cookie pan.
4. Then in the preheated oven, bake the dough 350 degrees F for approximately 12 minutes. Later, move the pan to a wire rack to cool at room temperature. Bon appétit!

Nutritions: Calories: 197, Fat: 15.8g, Carbs: 12.5g, Protein: 2.1g

133. VANILLA HALVAH FUDGE

PREPARATION: 10 MIN COOKING: CHILLING TIME SERVES: 1

INGREDIENTS

- 1/2 cup cocoa butter
- 1/2 cup tahini
- 8 dates pitted
- 1/4 teaspoon ground cloves
- A pinch grated nutmeg
- A coarse pinch salt
- 1 teaspoon vanilla extract

DIRECTIONS

1. Line a square baking pot with parchment paper.
2. Mix the materials until everything is well incorporated.
3. Scrape the batter into the parchment-lined pan. Put in your freezer until ready to serve. Bon appétit!

Nutritions: *Calories: 106, Fat: 9.8g, Carbs: 4.5g, Protein: 1.4g*

134. RAW CHOCOLATE MANGO PIE

PREPARATION: 10 MIN COOKING: CHILLING TIME SERVES: 1

INGREDIENTS

Avocado layer:
- 3 ripe avocados, pitted and peeled
- A pinch sea salt
- A bit ground anise
- 1/2 teaspoon vanilla paste
- 2 tablespoons coconut milk
- 5 tablespoons agave syrup
- 1/3 cup cocoa powder

Cream layer:
- 1/3 cup almond butter
- 1/2 cup coconut cream
- One medium mango, peeled
- 1/2 coconut flakes
- Two tablespoons agave syrup

DIRECTIONS

1. In your food processor, blend the avocado layer until smooth and uniform, reserve.
2. Then, blend the other layer in a separate bowl. Spoon the layers in a lightly oiled baking pan.
3. Move the cake to your freezer for about 3 hours. Store in your freezer. Bon appétit!

Nutritions: Calories: 196, Fat: 16.8g, Carbs: 14.1g, Protein: 1.8g

135. RAW RASPBERRY CHEESECAKE

PREPARATION: 15 MIN   COOKING: CHILLING TIME   SERVES: 1

INGREDIENTS

Crust:

- 2 cups almonds
- 1 cup fresh dates, pitted
- 1/4 teaspoon ground cinnamon

Filling:

- 2 cups raw cashews, drenched overnight and drained
- 14 oz. blackberries, frozen
- 1 tablespoon fresh lime juice
- 1/4 teaspoon crystallized ginger
- 1 can use coconut cream
- 8 fresh dates pitted

DIRECTIONS

1. Mix the crust ingredients using the food processor up until the mix comes together; press the crust into a lightly oiled spring form pan.
2. Then, blend the filling layer until completely smooth. Spoon the filling onto the crust, creating a flat surface with a spatula.
3. Transfer the cake to your freezer for around 3 hours. Store in your freezer.
4. Garnish with organic citrus peel. Bon appétit!

Nutritions: *Calories: 385, Fat: 22.9, Carbs: 41.1g, Protein: 10.8g*

136. MINI LEMON TARTS

PREPARATION: 15 MIN

COOKING: CHILLING TIME

SERVES: 1

INGREDIENTS

- 1 cup cashews
- 1 cup dates, pitted
- 1/2 cup coconut flakes
- 1/2 teaspoon anise, ground
- 3 lemons, freshly squeezed
- 1 cup coconut cream
- 2 tablespoons agave syrup

DIRECTIONS

1. Brush a muffin tin with nonstick cooking oil.
2. Blend the cashews, dates, coconut, and anise in your food processor or a high-speed blender. Press the crust into the peppered muffin tin.
3. Then, blend the lemon, coconut cream, and agave syrup. Spoon the cream into the muffin tin.
4. Store in your freezer. Bon appétit!

Nutritions: Calories: 257, Fat: 16.5, Carbs: 25.4g, Protein: 4g

137. FLUFFY COCONUT BLONDIES WITH RAISINS

PREPARATION: 30 MIN COOKING: 25 MIN SERVES: 1

INGREDIENTS

- 1 cup coconut flour
- 1 cup all-purpose flour
- 1/2 teaspoon baking powder
- 1/4 teaspoon salt
- 1 cup desiccated coconut, unsweetened
- 3/4 cup vegan butter, softened
- 1 ½ cups brown sugar
- 3 tablespoons applesauce
- 1/2 teaspoon vanilla extract
- 1/2 teaspoon ground anise
- 1 cup raisins, soaked for 15 minutes

DIRECTIONS

1. Begin by warming your oven to 400 degrees F. Brush a baking pan with nonstick cooking oil.
2. Carefully combine the flour, baking powder, salt, and coconut. In another bowl, mix the butter, sugar, applesauce, vanilla, and anise. Stir the butter mixture into the dry materials; stir to combine well.
3. Fold in the raisins. Swarm the batter into the prepared baking pan.
4. Bake for approximately 25 minutes or until it is set in the middle. Place the cake on a wire shelf to cool slightly.
5. Bon appétit!

Nutritions: *Calories: 365, Fat: 18.5, Carbs: 49g, Protein: 2.1g*

138. EASY CHOCOLATE SQUARES

PREPARATION: 20 MIN

COOKING: 60 MIN

SERVES: 1

INGREDIENTS

- 1 cup cashew butter
- 1 cup almond butter
- 1/4 cup coconut oil, melted
- 1/4 cup raw cacao powder
- 2 oz. dark chocolate
- 4 tablespoons agave syrup
- 1 teaspoon vanilla paste
- 1/4 teaspoon ground cinnamon
- 1/4 teaspoon ground cloves

DIRECTIONS

1. Process all the materials in your blender until uniform and smooth.
2. Scrape the batter into a parchment-lined baking sheet. Put it in the freezer. Wait for at least 1 hour to set.
3. Cut into squares and serve. Bon appétit!

Nutritions: Calories: 187, Fat: 13.8g, Carbs: 15.1g, Protein: 2.9g

139. FLUFFY COCONUT COOKIES

PREPARATION: 30 MIN

COOKING: 10 MIN

SERVES: 1

INGREDIENTS

- 1/2 cup oat flour
- 1/2 cup all-purpose flour
- 1/2 teaspoon baking soda
- A pinch of salt
- 1/4 teaspoon grated nutmeg
- 1/2 teaspoon ground cloves
- 1/2 teaspoon ground cinnamon
- 4 tablespoons coconut oil
- 2 tablespoons oat milk
- 1/2 cup coconut sugar
- 1/2 cup coconut flakes, unsweetened

DIRECTIONS

1. In a blending bowl, blend the flour, baking soda, and spices.
2. In another bowl, combine the coconut oil, oat milk, sugar, and coconut. Stir the wet mixture into the dry elements and stir until well combined.
3. Place the batter in your refrigerator for about 30 minutes. Shape the batter into small cookies and arrange them on a parchment-lined cookie pan.
4. Bake in the preheated oven at 330 degrees F for approximately 10 minutes. Move the pan to a wire rack to cool at room temperature. Bon appétit!

Nutritions: *Calories: 136, Fat: 7.3g, Carbs: 15.6g, Protein: 1.6g*

140. RAW WALNUT AND BERRY CAKE

PREPARATION: 10 MIN

COOKING: 0 MIN

SERVES: 1

INGREDIENTS

Crust:

- 1 ½ cup walnuts, ground
- 2 tablespoons maple syrup
- 1/4 cup raw cacao powder
- 1/4 teaspoon ground cinnamon
- A pinch of coarse salt
- A bit of freshly grated nutmeg

Berry layer:

- 6 cups mixed berries
- 2 frozen bananas
- 1/2 cup agave syrup

DIRECTIONS

1. Blend the crust ingredients using the food processor until the mixture comes together; press the crust into a lightly oiled baking pan.
2. Then, blend the berry layer. Spoon the berry layer onto the crust, creating a flat surface with a spatula.
3. Transfer the cake to the freezer for about 3 hours. Store in your freezer. Bon appétit!

Nutritions: Calories: 244, Fat: 10.2g, Carbs: 39g, Protein: 3.8g

141. CHOCOLATE DREAM BALLS

PREPARATION: 10 MIN

COOKING: 0 MIN

SERVES: 1

INGREDIENTS

- 3 tablespoons cocoa powder
- 8 fresh dates pitted and soaked for 15 minutes
- 2 tablespoons tahini, at room temperature
- 1/2 teaspoon ground cinnamon
- 1/2 cup vegan chocolate, broken into chunks
- One tablespoon coconut oil, at room temperature

DIRECTIONS

1. Add the cocoa powder, dates, tahini, and cinnamon to the bowl of your food processor. Process until the mixture forms a ball.
2. Use a cookie scoop to piece the mixture into 1- oz. portions. Roll the balls and refrigerate them for at least 30 minutes.
3. Meanwhile, microwave the chocolate until melted; add in the coconut oil and whisk to combine well.
4. Dip the chocolate balls in the layer and store them in your refrigerator until ready to serve. Bon appétit!

Nutritions: *Calories: 107, Fat: 7.2g, Carbs: 10.8g, Protein: 1.8g*

142. LAST MINUTE MACAROONS

PREPARATION: 5 MIN

COOKING: 10 MIN

SERVES: 1

INGREDIENTS

- 3 cups coconut flakes, sweetened
- 9 oz. canned coconut milk, sweetened
- 1 teaspoon ground anise
- 1 teaspoon vanilla extract

DIRECTIONS

1. Head start by warming your oven to 400 degrees F. Line the cookie sheets with parchment paper.
2. Thoroughly combine all the ingredients until everything is well incorporated.
3. Use a cookie scoop to drop mounds of the batter onto the prepared cookie sheets.
4. Bake for about 12 to 15 minutes.
5. Wait until they are lightly browned. Bon appétit!

Nutritions: Calories: 125, Fat: 7.2g, Carbs: 14.3g, Protein: 1.1g

143. OLD-FASHIONED RATAFIAS

PREPARATION: 5 MIN | COOKING: 15 MIN | SERVES: 1

INGREDIENTS

- 2 oz. all-purpose flour
- 2 oz. almond flour
- 1 teaspoon baking powder
- 2 tablespoons applesauce
- 5 oz. caster sugar
- 1(½-oz.) vegan butter
- 4 drops of ratafia essence

DIRECTIONS

1. Start by warming your oven to 330 degrees F. Line a cookie sheet with parchment paper.
2. Thoroughly combine all the ingredients until everything is well incorporated.
3. Use a cookie scoop to drop mounds of the batter onto the prepared cookie sheet.
4. Bake for about 12 to 15 minutes.
5. Wait until they are lightly browned. Bon appétit!

Nutritions: *Calories: 272, Fat: 16.2g, Carbs: 28.6g, Protein: 5.8g*

CONCLUSION

You had reached the end of this book. You now know a lot about the Optavia Diet and even about recipes for this diet. I do hope you had already cooked several recipes. Will you agree with me that they are delicious?

Let me just point out some essential items once again to help you remember and value it.

The Optavia Diet can be effectively used for rapid weight loss compared to other plans simply because of the offer made by lean and green meals and its few calories.

Based on the U.S. News and World Report, it listed Optavia on the number 2 position on the best diet for rapid weight loss. They tied with Keto, Atkins, and Weight Watchers.

However, the 2019 U.S. News and World Report Best Diets positioned the Optavia Diet in the number 31 in the list of Best Diets overall and graded it as 2.7/5.

Optavia doesn't require much-exerted energy compared to its competitors such as Weight Watchers (here, you will have to master a system of points) or Keto (here, you must assess and closely track macronutrients).

The coaching component of Optavia compared to Jenny Craig and Weight Watchers, which urge users to register for meetups to get the necessary support.

But because of the highly processed nature of most of the foods available in the Optavia diet, it could pose a threat or challenge compared to the variety of whole, fresh foods you can consume in more self-sustaining plans such as Atkins.

The Optavia diet enables weight loss through one-on-one coaching, low carb homemade meals, and low-calorie prepackaged diets.

Although the initial 5&1 Plan is quite limiting, the 3&3 maintenance phase enables fewer processed snacks and a wider variety of food, making it easier to lose weight and adhere to the program for sustenance in the long term.

Nevertheless, the diet is repetitive, costly, and doesn't cover all dietary needs. Another point is that extended calorie restriction may lead to nutrient deficiencies and other risky health concerns.

Although the program promotes fat loss and short-term weight loss, further research is required to evaluate the level of lifestyle changes it needs for long-term success.

If you ever succeed on the structure and need to get fit rapidly, the Optavia Diet could be a solid match for you.

Before you start any feast substitution dict, cautiously consider whether you can sensibly tail it, choose how much cash you can contribute, and decide the level of craving and interference in your social routine that you feel good about.

If you ever will settle on Optavia and prevail with your transient weight loss objectives, ensure you become taught about smart dieting to keep the weight in the long-term because that is the common mishap of people who follow this diet. Always maintain.

It had been a long journey for finding the most appropriate diet or learning recipes that you may use. You may continue with your quest on the Optavia Diet.

CPSIA information can be obtained
at www.ICGtesting.com
Printed in the USA
LVHW060914090121
675633LV00066B/33

9 781801 540902